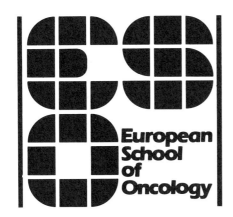

Monographs

Series Editor: U.Veronesi

L. Tomatis (Ed.)

Air Pollution and Human Cancer

With 7 Figures and 10 Tables

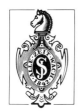

Springer-Verlag Berlin Heidelberg New York
London Paris Tokyo Hong Kong Barcelona

Lorenzo Tomatis

International Agency for Research on Cancer
150, cours Albert-Thomas
69372 Lyon Cedex 08, France

The European School of Oncology gratefully acknowledges the educational grant for the production of this monograph received from SNAM, Italy

ISBN 3-540-52901-2 Springer-Verlag Berlin Heidelberg New York
ISBN 0-387-52901-2 Springer-Verlag New York Berlin Heidelberg

Library of Congress Cataloging-in-Publication Data
Air pollution and human cancer / L. Tomatis (ed.) p. cm.–(Monographs / European School of Oncology) ISBN 3-540-52901-2 (alk. paper).–ISBN 0-387-52901-2 (alk. paper) 1. Carcinogenesis. 2. Air–Pollution–Health aspects. I. Tomatis, L. II. Series: Monographs (European School of Oncology) [DNLM: 1. Air Pollutants–adverse effects. 2. Air Pollution. 3. Neoplasms–etiology. QZ 202 A298] RC268.5.A37 1990 616.99'4071–dc20 DNLM/DLC for Library of Congress 90-10135 CIP

© Springer-Verlag Berlin Heidelberg 1990
Printed in Germany

The use of general descriptive names, registered names, trademarks, etc. in this publication does not imply, even in the absence of a specific statement, that such names are exempt from the relevant protective laws and regulations and therefore free for general use.

Product Liability: The publisher can give no guarantee for information about drug dosage and application thereof contained in this book. In every individual case the respective user must check its accuracy by consulting other pharmaceutical literature.

Printing: Druckhaus Beltz, Hemsbach/Bergstr.; Bookbinding: J. Schäffer GmbH & Co. KG, Grünstadt
2123/3145-543210 – Printed on acid-free paper

Foreword

The European School of Oncology came into existence to respond to a need for information, education and training in the field of the diagnosis and treatment of cancer. There are two main reasons why such an initiative was considered necessary. Firstly, the teaching of oncology requires a rigorously multidisciplinary approach which is difficult for the Universities to put into practice since their system is mainly disciplinary orientated. Secondly, the rate of technological development that impinges on the diagnosis and treatment of cancer has been so rapid that it is not an easy task for medical faculties to adapt their curricula flexibly.

With its residential courses for organ pathologies and the seminars on new techniques (laser, monoclonal antibodies, imaging techniques etc.) or on the principal therapeutic controversies (conservative or mutilating surgery, primary or adjuvant chemotherapy) radiotherapy alone or integrated), it is the ambition of the European School of Oncology to fill a cultural and scientific gap and, thereby, create a bridge between the University and Industry and between these two and daily medical practice.

One of the more recent initiatives of ESO has been the institution of permanent study groups, also called task forces, where a limited number of leading experts are invited to meet once a year with the aim of defining the state of the art and possibly reaching a consensus on future developments in specific fields of oncology.

The ESO Monograph series was designed with the specific purpose of disseminating the results of these study group meetings, and providing concise and updated reviews of the topic discussed.

It was decided to keep the layout relatively simple, in order to restrict the costs and make the monographs available in the shortest possible time, thus overcoming a common problem in medical literature: that of the material being outdated even before publication.

UMBERTO VERONESI
Chairman Scientific Committee
European School of Oncology

Contents

Air Pollution and Cancer: An Old and New Problem

Lorenzo Tomatis

International Agency for Research on Cancer, 150, cours Albert-Thomas, 69372 Lyon Cedex 08, France

The history of mankind can be divided into 3 periods: the period of hunters-gatherers, the period that followed the agricultural revolution and the period that followed industrialisation. In his latest book, McKeown [1] observed that "in the first period there was no effective control either on the environment or on reproduction; in the second period there was some control on the environment but not on reproduction and in the third period there was further control on the environment and, for the first time, on reproduction but there was insufficient control on the conditions of life created by industrialisation."

McKeown's definition of the third period should perhaps be slightly altered, to read "further control but also further abuse of the environment", since, in fact, having imposed ourselves on the environment, we are at present concerned with the difficulty or the incapacity to control or reverse the modifications we have induced.

Air pollution is certainly not a new phenomenon. Indoor pollution was probably experienced by the inhabitants of caves and of primitive houses, which had no or insufficient evacuation of fumes, and natural phenomena like volcanic eruptions and the accidental or voluntary burning of woods and forests have certainly contributed to the emission of pollutants into the air since time immemorial.

There is little doubt, however, that air pollution has increased recently; the pollution of air near certain industrial plants and in large cities is one of the alterations to human existence brought about by industrialisation. René Dubos [2] observed that, although air pollution is an old phenomenon, the introduction of more of the same and new pollutants on a large scale has recently transformed it into an important health problem. Trends in estimated emissions of some of the most important air pollutants have been calculated for the world [3] and for individual countries [4]. These show that air pollution has become a planetary problem, and there is now no area of the earth that has been spared the presence and consequences of air pollution, as pollutants can cause damage far away from their point of emission into the atmosphere [5].

This monograph will address the possible association between air pollution and human cancer and touches only briefly and marginally on adverse effects other than cancer. Most attention is paid to the sources of and exposure to outdoor pollutants, although, clearly, external pollutants almost inevitably end up indoors and add to those generated by indoor sources. Exposures to environmental tobacco smoke (passive smoking) and to radon are therefore mentioned only briefly. Similarly, sources and routes of exposure other than air and through air, e.g., the presence of polycyclic aromatic hydrocarbons in certain foods, are only mentioned.

Air pollution may have many indirect health effects which are not covered in this volume, including those associated with the increased mobilisation of metals, such as aluminium, cadmium and mercury, due to the increasing acidification of soil and waters.

Evidence for Severe Acute Effects

The worst effects of air pollution were seen in the U.K., probably due to the combination of early introduction of coal for heating and cooking purposes and early and rapid spread of industries, in a country where climatic conditions favour the formation of smog. In 1965, R. Dubos [2] quoted an anecdote about William Harvey, who performed an autopsy on the centenarian "Old Parr" and concluded that he had probably died because he was exposed to the heavily polluted air of London after having lived all his life in the country. John Evelyn [6] described the filthy air of London in 1661 and associated the exposure to the thick London smog with a variety of health problems.

More recently, the severe adverse effects that can be caused by air pollution were demonstrated dramatically by a series of disasters, the best known of which are those that occurred in Liège, Belgium, in 1930, in Donora, Pennsylvania, in 1948 and in London in the winter of 1952 [7,8]. In Belgium, 63 people died following what was called a "smog incident". In Donora, due to an infrequent (but not exceptional) phenomenon of thermal inversion, the smog persisted and accumulated for several days, causing severe health effects in almost 600 inhabitants, of whom 17 died. In London, in a little over a week of the winter of 1952, more than 4,000 people died due to the heavy smog. It was this last episode that finally triggered the introduction of severe measures to reduce air pollution. The Clean Air Act was approved and rigidly enforced in the U.K. in 1956, with subsequent considerable reduction in air pollution in London and several other large cities. There is some evidence that further decreases in the present level of air pollution, in particular of suspended particulates, in cities like London could probably contribute to reducing mortality further [9].

A 10-year follow-up of the residents of Donora indicates higher mortality and morbidity among people who were exposed during the smog episode as compared with non-exposed persons [10]. While this increase might, to a considerable extent, be attributable to a worsening of pre-existing heart and lung conditions, there is some evidence of increased morbidity among exposed individuals who had no pre-existing heart or lung conditions.

The Effects of (Relatively) Low Levels of Exposure

Adverse effects due to low levels of exposure may be much more difficult to ascertain, especially in the case of long-term chronic effects, such as cancer.

In many instances, cancer is the result of a subjectively symptomless sequence and accumulation of pathological events which may begin early in life or even prenatally. This is one important reason why exposures involving entire populations, from the youngest to the oldest age groups, are of particular public health concern. On the one hand, even low levels of exposure may be acutely harmful to individuals who are particularly fragile with regard to health effects - like the very young and the very old; on the other hand, even low exposure levels may be harmful in the long run, and the more so the longer the duration of exposure.

As will be better explained in Chapters 2 and 3, much progress has been made in the development of analytical methods to detect chemicals in our environment. Specific chemicals can now be detected at levels lower by orders of magnitude than those that could be detected 20 years ago. Progress in toxicology and in the understanding of the mechanisms of carcinogenesis has not, however, kept the same pace. One of the main unresolved problems is the assessment of risks related to very low levels of exposure (as low as the levels of detectability of the available analytical methods) to a toxic agent. The problem is amplified by the fact that people are always exposed to several agents at the same time.

This paradoxical situation - that technological progress, instead of improving our decision-making capacity, has apparently widened our uncertainties - will hopefully be resolved with the development and continuous improvement of methods for the biological monitoring of individual exposures.

The recent worsening of the problem of air pollution has both quantitative and qualitative components: chemical pollutants that occurred at limited concentrations or in limited areas now occur in greater amounts and are more widespread, and newly synthesised chemical compounds are being emitted. The accumulation of these 2 components began during the last century and has not ceased. Furthermore, photochemical reactions in the atmosphere may engender new chemical species.

Two major types of air pollution have been described: a "reducing" form, often called "London smog", resulting mainly from the incomplete combustion of coal and oil, the main components of which are soots, sulphur dioxide, nitrogen oxides and sulphuric acids; and an "oxidising" form, often called "Los Angeles smog", the main components of which are carbon monoxide, hydrocarbons and photochemical decomposition products. The urban atmosphere in which various particulates and pollutant gases accumulate, react and interreact under the influence of sunlight, has been described as "a giant chemical reactor" [11].

Chemical agents that were present in the environment before the industrial revolution began - such as asbestos and certain metals - have been exploited on a massive scale only since the last century but increasingly during the present one. While these agents have been present for a long time, it is only since their massive industrial use that they have become a conspicuous source of hazardous exposure of both occupational groups and the general population.

Asbestos is found almost over the entire planet. For example, Japan, where there was no domestic production of asbestos, began to import it in growing quantities in the 1950s. A retrospective survey on the presence of asbestiform bodies in the lungs of the general population showed an impressive correlation between the increased importation and increase in the percentage of individuals with these bodies [12]. Japan is probably the only country in which a specific law allows compensation of pollution-related health damage. At the beginning of 1988, there were over 100,000 individuals in Japan receiving compensation for diseases related to air pollution [13].

About 60 million tons of bitumens are produced worldwide annually [14], most of which is used to pave roads and airstrips and for roofing. Although we know that bitumens contain several carcinogens/mutagens, we have no way of knowing whether the millions of tons used every year contribute in any way to

our load of carcinogens. Similar considerations could be applied to rubber, as more than half of the 13 million tons (1980) produced annually is used in tyres [15], a large part of which is rubbed off onto our bitumen-paved roads.

A more detailed account of the spectrum of hazardous inorganic and organic, natural and anthropogenic pollutants discharged into the atmosphere, and of those that are formed as a consequence of the dynamics of atmospheric reactions and photochemical transformations, is given in Chapter 2 (see also [16]). While the first experimental evidence that urban air pollutants are carcinogenic was produced half a century ago [17,18], we are still far from identifying all of the genotoxic and non-genotoxic compounds present in ambient air, in spite of the spectacular progress made in identification procedures [19].

Lung Cancer

Most studies on the carcinogenicity of air pollution have focussed on the possible association with cancer of the lung, and only a few have addressed cancers at other sites. The emphasis on lung cancer derives naturally from the fact that exposure to air pollutants is primarily via the respiratory tract. Furthermore, the lung is one of the preferred target organs for those agents and complex exposures that have been established as carcinogenic to humans [20]. While tobacco smoke is by far the most important lung carcinogen, a causal association with lung cancer has been demonstrated for 11 other carcinogenic agents and 6 complex exposures.

Carcinogens to which exposure occurs mainly by inhalation may also induce tumours at sites other than the respiratory tract; for instance, bladder and pancreatic cancers, and possibly liver and kidney cancers, are causally related to the inhalation of tobacco smoke. Air pollutants may also be ingested or penetrate the skin [21-23].

While this monograph is clearly focussed on cancer, it must be remembered that air pollutants also have subchronic and chronic adverse effects other than cancer. Since an increased frequency of respiratory tract diseases is observed most often in children [24], it is relevant that lower respiratory infections early in life are linked to an increased risk of chronic bronchitis during adult life [25]. Some experimental results point to other possible toxic effects: a variety of carcinogenic and non-carcinogenic polycyclic hydrocarbons that are air pollutants can promote the formation of arteriosclerotic plaques [26].

An accurate evaluation of the role of outdoor air pollution in increasing the risk for lung cancer is made particularly arduous because of confounding by other carcinogenic exposures, such as active and passive smoking, a number of occupational exposures, radon gas and other indoor pollutants. (The role of indoor pollutants should be dealt with in a separate monograph or, preferably, in a subsequent, expanded version of the present one.) In addition, air pollutants may interact with other carcinogens, as is the case for tobacco smoke with asbestos and with radon.

Recent experimental results provide the basis for methods to discriminate between the "spontaneous" lung and liver tumours and those induced by chemical agents [27,28]. It may therefore soon become possible to understand the extent to which different aetiological agents concur, additively or multiplicatively, to increase the risk of cancer of the lung and other sites, and, therefore, to calculate accurately the risks attributable to combined exposures to specific agents.

Most of the studies on the association between air pollution and lung cancer have focussed on the role of the urban environment. As a rule, mortality rates for lung cancer are higher in large cities and are inversely correlated to the density of the population [29]. Although the highest urban:rural ratio for lung cancer was observed where emissions from the burning of coal for domestic purposes and industrial emissions coexisted for the longest time, urban air pollution is not limited to industrialised countries. The highest concentrations of suspended particulate matter, sulphur dioxide and smoke have, in fact, been recorded in large cities in developing countries [30,31]. In China, for instance, although considerable efforts are being made to reduce emissions, levels of particulates in urban areas and in areas around industrial settings are still very high [32]. The use of smoky coals may result in particularly severe pollution of indoor air: the highest incidence of lung tumours in the world has been reported in women of a region in China who are exposed in their houses to smoke from coal used for cooking and heating. Massive urbanisation in association with poverty, resulting in a huge increase in urban pollution and poor hygiene, is a growing problem in developing countries. In 1965, 17% of the total population of developing countries with low incomes lived in large cities; in 1987, this was the case for 30% of the population [33]. The concentrations of particulate matter and of sulphur dioxide are high in certain large cities in developing countries [3], but some of the worst pollution levels have been observed in Poland, where recent data suggest that the levels of exposure of the general population to air pollutants in certain regions are comparable to the highest ever observed in specific hazardous occupations (see this volume).

Interactions Between Carcinogenic Agents

It is in situations of heavy air pollution that interactions between air pollution and carcinogenic exposures, such as smoking and certain occupational exposures, can best be demonstrated. Interaction between carcinogens in increasing the risk of lung cancer is well documented in the case of asbestos and tobacco smoking, which appear to interact multiplicatively [34,35], and there is convincing evidence of an additive (and perhaps multiplicative) effect between radiation and tobacco smoke [36]. In a case-control study, air pollution appeared to contribute to a significant increase in the risk of lung cancer among smokers who had had carcinogenic occupational exposures [37,38]. This finding contrasts with the results of case-control studies in which excesses of lung cancer could be explained entirely (or almost entirely) by smoking habits and occupation [39,40], although a more recent study points to an independent role of air pollution in increasing the risk of lung cancer [41]. A number of studies indicate an increased lung cancer risk in passive smokers, that is, individuals who are exposed to tobacco smoke released into the ambient air by smokers [42]. The strongest argument to support the epidemiological findings is that persons exposed to environmental tobacco smoke are exposed to a chemical mixture containing known carcinogens, that is, substances known to cause cancer in smokers. Since there is a quantitative, non-threshold dose-response relationship in active smokers, one can reasonably conclude that exposure to environmental tobacco smoke must also increase the risk of cancer [36]. It is tempting to compare exposure to air pollution to exposure to environmental tobacco smoke and to see it as a particular type of air pollution. Urban air and the air in the proximity of certain factories contain substances that have been shown to be carcinogenic at exposure levels that can occur in occupational environments. Jedrychowski et al. [43] found that the joint action of air pollution, smoking and occupational exposures is well described by a multiplicative model.

The Problems of Ozone

Ozone can exert both deleterious and beneficial effects - acting as a significant pollutant locally, while providing a valuable photochemical screen against excess ultra-violet radiation at high altitudes. Ozone is a highly reactive, powerful oxidant which can react with virtually any class of biological substance, resulting in rapid reactions, particularly in the cells, fluids and tissues lining the respiratory tract. Its 2 major effects are alterations (usually impairment) in the mechanical functions of the lung, often accompanied by respiratory symptoms, and structural injury to or functional impairment of specific types of cells in the respiratory tract [16,44,45]. The primary source of excess tropospheric ozone is reactions between the hydrocarbons and oxides of nitrogen emitted from the burning of fossil fuels. It may also be produced biogenically from the reaction between nitric oxide made by soil microbes and terpenes and other hydrocarbons released from trees. The maximal ozone concentrations that are attained in polluted atmospheres are dependent on the absolute concentrations of volatile organic compounds and nitrogen oxides as well as their ratio [11,16,46,47]. The chlorinated fluorocarbons, which are widely used as refrigerants and aerosol propellants, are long-lived atmospheric pollutants that have been implicated in the dramatic decreases in atmospheric ozone levels. Ozone absorbs ultra-violet radiation in the B region (280-320 nm) which would otherwise reach the earth's surface, and its depletion may adversely affect human health. Both epidemiological studies and the results of tests with animal models link squamous-cell and basal-cell skin cancers to exposure to ultra-violet radiation, and there is convincing evidence that it contributes to an increase in the risk of malignant melanomas. It is, therefore, possible that increased radiation may generate an increased risk of pigmented and non-pigmented skin tumours [3]. Increased radiation may also have deleterious effects on plants, marine organisms and synthetic materials [11,46,47].

The Greenhouse Effect and Acid Rain

Atmospheric emissions in both developing and developed (industrialised) countries can have regional and global consequences, as evidenced by the depletion of the ozone layer mentioned above, by the increasing problems related to acid rain and by the greenhouse effect, even though the mechanisms, rate and extent of possible damage remain to be elucidated or modelled.

There is increasing evidence that the composition of the atmosphere is changing, due to rising levels of pollutants and "greenhouse" gases such as carbon dioxide, nitrous oxide, methane and the chlorofluorocarbons, which have regional and global consequences on the production of acid rain, the greenhouse effect and depletion of the ozone layer by mechanisms currently not fully defined [30,46,47]. In the case of acid rain, acidic substances and their precursors are formed when fossil fuels are burnt to generate power and provide transportation. Although there are some natural sources of the principal precursors (the oxides of sulphur and nitrogen), these are relatively minor compared to emissions from smelters, power plants and vehicles in industrialised regions. However, the routes by which the oxides of nitrogen and sulphur are formed, undergo chemical transformation and are eventually removed from the atmosphere, are very complex and have not been completely elucidated [48,49].

REFERENCES

1   McKeown Th: The Origins of Human Disease. Basil Blackwell, Oxford 1988

2   Dubos R: Man Adapting. Yale University Press, Yale 1965

3   UNEP Environmental Data Report 1989-1990. Basil Blackwell Inc Publ, Cambridge, MA, USA, 1989

4   Bocola W and Cirillo MC: Air pollutant emissions by combustion processes in Italy. Atmosph Environ 1989 (23 No 1):17-24

5   Derwent D: A better way to control pollution. Nature 1988 (331):575-578

6   Evelyn J: The Inconvenience of the Air and Smoke of London Dissipated. London 1661 (cited by R. Dubos, 1965)

7   Lawther PJ, Martin A and Wilkins ET: Epidemiology of air pollution. WHO PH paper No 15, 1962

8   Wilkins ET: Air pollution and the London fog of December 1952. J Roy San Inst 1954 (74):1-21

9   Schwartz J and Marcus A: Mortality and air pollution in London: A time series analysis. Am J Epidem 1990 (131):185-194

10   Ciocco A and Thompson D: A follow-up of Donora ten years after. Amer J Publ Hlth 1961 (51):155-164

11   Seinfeld JH: Urban air pollution: State of the Science. Science 1989 (243):745-752

12   Shishido S, Iwai K and Tukagoshi K: Incidence of ferruginous bodies in the lungs during a 45-year period and mineralogical analysis of the core fibres and uncoated fibres. In: Bignon J, Peto J and Saracci R (eds) Non-Occupational Exposure to Mineral Fibres. IARC Scientific Publications Series No 90. International Agency for Research on Cancer, Lyon 1989 pp 229-238

13   Quality of the Environment in Japan. Environment Agency. Government of Japan, 1988

14   IARC Monograph on the Evaluation of Carcinogenic Risks to Humans, Vol 35: Polynuclear Aromatic Compounds, Part 4, Bitumens, Coal-Tars and Derived Products, Shale-Oils and Soots. International Agency for Research on Cancer, Lyon 1985

15   IARC Monograph on the Evaluation of Carcinogenic Risks to Humans, Vol 28: The Rubber Industry. International Agency for Research on Cancer, Lyon 1982

16   World Health Organization: Air Quality Guidelines for Europe. WHO Regional Publications. European Series No 23, Copenhagen 1987 pp 315-326

17   Leiter J, Shimkin MB and Shear MJ: Production of subcutaneous sarcomas in mice with tars extracted from atmospheric dusts. JNCI 1942 (3):155-165

18   Leiter J and Shear MJ: Production of tumors in mice with tars from city air dusts. JNCI 1942 (3):167-174

19   Schuetzle D and Daisey JM: Identification of genotoxic agents in complex mixtures of air pollutants. In: Waters MD, Nesnow S, Lewtas J, Moore MM and Daniel FB (eds) Short-Term Bioassays in the Analysis of Complex Environmental Mixtures, VI. Plenum Press, New York 1990

20   Tomatis L, Aitio A, Shuker L and Wilbourn J: Human carcinogens so far identified. Jpn J Cancer Res 1989 (80):795-807

21   Sellers Storer J, DeLeon I, Millikan LE, Laseter JL and Griffing C: Human absorption of coal-tar products. Arch Dermatol 1984 (120):874-877

22   Jongeneelen FJ, Leijdekkers ChM and Henderson PTh: Urinary excretion of 3-hydroxy-benzo(a)pyrene after percutaneous penetration and oral absorption of benzo(a)pyrene in rats. Cancer Letters 1984 (25):195-201

23   Yang JJ, Roy TA and Mackerer CR: Percutaneous absorption of anthracene in the rat: comparison of in vivo and in vitro results. Toxicol and Indus Hlth 1986 (2):79-84

24   Goren A, Brenner S and Hellmann S: Cross-sectional health study in polluted and nonpolluted agricultural settlements in Israel. Environ Hlth 1988 (46):107-119

25   Barker DJP, Osmond C and Law CM: The intrauterine and early postnatal origins of cardiovascular disease and chronic bronchitis. J Epidemiol Comm Hlth 1989 (43):237-240

26   Penn A and Snyder C: Arterosclerotic plaque development is "promoted" by polynuclear aromatic hydrocarbons. Carcinogenesis 1989 (9):2185-2189

27   Wiseman RW, Stowers SJ, Miller EC, Anderson MW and Miller JA: Activating mutations of the c-Ha-ras protooncogene in chemically induced hepatomas of the male B6C3F1 mouse. Proc Natl Acad Sci USA 1986 (83):5825-5829

28   You M, Candrian U, Maronpot RR, Stoner GD and Anderson MW: Activation of the Ki-ras protooncogene in spontaneously occurring and

chemically induced lung tumours of the strain A mice. Proc Natl Acad Sci USA 1989 (86):3074-3079

29 Muir CS, Waterhouse J, Mack T, Powell J and Whelan S (eds) Cancer Incidence in Five Continents, Vol V. IARC Scientific Publications no. 88, Lyon 1987

30 Bennett BG, Kretzschmar JG, Akland GG and Dekoning HW: Urban air pollution worldwide. Environ Sci Technol 1985 (19):298-304

31 Böhm GM, Nascimento Saldiva PH, Goncalves Pasqualucci CA, Massad E, De Arruda Martins M, Araujo Zin W, Veras Cardoso W, Martins Pereira Criado P, Komatsuzaki M, Sakae RS, Negri EM, Lemos M, Del Monte Capelozzi V, Crestana C and Da Silva R: Biological effects of air pollution in Sao Paulo and Cubatao. Environmental Res 1989 (49):208-216

32 Assessment of Urban air quality. UNEP/WHO 1988

33 World Development Report 1989, Oxford University Press 1989

34 Hammond EC, Selikoff JJ, Seidman H: Asbestos exposure, cigarette smoking and death rates. Ann NY Acad Sciences 1979 (330):473-490

35 Saracci R: The interactions of tobacco smoking and other agents in cancer etiology. Epidemiol Rev 1987 (9):175-193

36 Cancer: Causes, occurrence and control. IARC 1990

37 Vena JE: Air pollution as a risk factor in lung cancer. Am J Epidemiol 1982 (116):42-56

38 Winkelstein W Jr and Levin LI: Air pollution and cancer. Rev in Cancer Epidemiol 1983 (2):211-239

39 Haenszel W, Loveland DB and Sirken MG: Lung cancer mortality as related to residence and smoking histories. JNCI 1962 (28):947-1001

40 Pike MC, Jing JS, Rosario IP, Henderson BE and Menck HR: Occupation: explanation of an apparent air pollution related localized excess of lung cancer in Los Angeles County. In: Breslow N and Whittemore A (eds) Energy and Health. SIAM, Philadelphia PA 1979 pp 3-16

41 Buffler A, Cooper P, Stonnett S, Contant Ch, Shirts S, Hardy J, Agu U, Gehan B, Buraj K: Air pollution and lung cancer mortality in Hanis County, Texas, 1979-1981. J Epidemiol 1988 (128):683-699

42 Saracci R and Riboli E: Passive smoking and lung cancer: current evidence and ongoing studies at the International Agency for Research on Cancer. Mutation Res 1989 (222):117-127

43 Jedrychowski W, Becher H, Wahrendorf J and Basa-Cierpalek Z: A case-control study of lung cancer with special reference to the effect of air pollution in Poland. J Epidemiol Comm Hlth 1989 (in press)

44 Tilton BE: Health effects of tropospheric ozone. Environ Sci Technol 1989 (23):254-263

45 US Environmental Protection Agency: Air quality criteria for ozone and other photochemical oxidants. 4 volumes. Report No. EPA-600/8-84-02F. Washington, DC 1986

46 Ember LR, Layman PL, Lepkowski W and Zurer PS: Tending the global commons. Chem Eng News 1989 (Nov 4):14-64

47 McElroy MB and Salawitch RJ: Changing composition of the global stratosphere. Science 1989 (243):763-770

48 Schwartz SE: Acid decomposition: Unraveling a regional phenomenon. Science 1989 (243):753-763

49 Anon: Reducing acid rain: Continuation of the Pimental Report. Environ Sci Technol 1985 (29):439-440

Sources, Nature and Levels of Air Pollutants

Lawrence Fishbein

ILSI-Risk Science Institute, Washington, DC 20036, U.S.A.

A broad spectrum of potentially toxic chemicals spanning many inorganic and organic structural categories, is released into local, regional and global atmospheres from both natural as well as anthropogenic sources and from both industrialised and developing countries [1-9]. In one data base compilation, more than 2,800 atmospheric compounds were identified of which slightly more than 300 (about 11%) have been bioassayed [1]. The introduction of toxicants into the atmosphere may be direct via the inadvertent or deliberate release from a particular mobile or stationary source, or indirectly as a consequence of initial discharge or disposal of chemicals to other environmental media, such as water or soil. Hazardous pollutants may be accidentally released into ambient air or via escape of raw materials or finished products at their manufacturing site (e.g., release of methyl isocyanate in Bohpal, India), or by a chemical spill resulting from a transportation mishap such as a truck, cargo train derailment and/or barge spillage or collision. Many toxicants are accidentally released from the thousands of chemical facilities and numerous small businesses such as dry cleaning establishments and service stations. Nitrogen oxides, carbon monoxide and volatile organic chemicals (VOCs) (e.g., benzene, toluene and xylene) have been identified in many instances to be primarily related to tailpipe emission and in the case of VOCs to exposure to emissions from petrol stations as well [1-9]. Pollutants also occur in the atmosphere as a result of myriad atmospheric reactions and photochemical transformations, and the chemical species present vary with precursor pollutants, altitude, season and location [3-5]. Urban areas are increasingly plagued with air pollution from complex mixtures of gases and particles with condensed organic matter emitted primarily from the combustion of fossil fuels (e.g., oil, coal, petrol, diesel fuel) from vehicle, industrial and power sources as well as from vegetative sources (e.g., wood, plant, and materials) [2-4,10-12]. In addition, many pollutants originating in outdoor air (e.g., carbon monoxide, nitrogen dioxide, formaldehyde, hydrocarbons, VOCs, pesticides, metals) are believed to contribute substantially to indoor air pollution, which is increasingly recognised as a potentially significant public health problem [11,12]. More than 65,000 chemicals are used in commerce in the industrialised nations of the world. Many of these substances, e.g., industrial solvents, VOCs, polychlorinated biphenyls, pesticides, and aerosol products containing volatile propellants and active ingredients, are emitted directly or indirectly because of man's activities [13].

Physical Properties, Stability, Fate, Transformation and Transport

Following emission into the atmosphere, individual pollutants possess characteristic residence times (life times) which are a function of source parameters as well as the physical and chemical properties of the pollutant and/or their photochemical reactivity [3-5,7,13].

Although the earth's atmosphere is composed of principally inert molecules or chemically reducing gases such as nitrogen, hydrogen and methane, the atmosphere acts as an oxidative system because of its *overall* composition and the relative chemical reactivity of natural atmospheric constituents and/or contaminants. The more chemically reactive species in the atmosphere include: atomic oxygen, ozone, hydroxyl and other free radicals (e.g., HO_2, CH_3O_2), peroxides (H_2O_2, CH_3O_2H), nitrogen oxides, sulphur oxides and wide variety of acidic and basic species. Hence a broad spectrum of natural and anthropogenic pollutants, once emitted into ambient air, can be potentially converted at various rates into species characterised by higher chemical oxidation states than their precursor substances. The fate of toxic air pollutants is determined by a variety of physical chemical and/or photochemical processes occurring in the atmosphere during their residence time in this environmental compartment. In addition to the concern of the direct action of atmospheric pollutants on human health, atmospheric input is believed to be the predominant source for a number of toxic pollutants in lakes and streams. For instance, 60-90% of the polychlorinated biphenyl (PCB) burden in the Great Lakes in the United States has been estimated to originate from the atmosphere [3-5,7,13].

The majority of emission sources release pollutants into the atmosphere close to or directly upon the earth's surface, and the height at which pollutants are released will determine the distance of their travel before their contact with the ground or another receptor surface [13]. It is important for an assessment of the impact of atmosphere emission sources on human health (as well as natural ecosystems) to quantify emissions to the extent possible, both spatially and temporally. Physical processes will act on pollutants immediately following their release from an emission source. This initial interaction is dependent on factors including the actual configuration of the emission source (area, height above the surrounding terrain) and initial buoyancy conditions [3,13]. Following emission, pollutants generally enter into a mixing layer in the lower region of the troposphere (which typically extends to 1-2 km during the day and a few hundred meters in the evening), where the pollutants circulate and disperse vertically and horizontally, promoting intimate contact between vapour-phase and aerosol-associated constituents [3,13]. This initial, important,

direct contact ultimately results in chemical transformations of pollutants near their source while their concentrations are still relatively high and precedes extensive dilution [13]. Diffusion and transport processes occur simultaneously in the atmosphere. Pollution transport is dependent on air mass circulations effected by local, regional or global forces. Dispersion represents the combination of transport and diffusion processes. Compared to the major pollutants of an inorganic nature (e.g., SO_2, NO_2, CO_2), considerably less is known of the movement and behaviour of many of the trace organic contaminants in the atmosphere [3-5,7,13].

During transport and diffusion through the atmosphere, many toxic pollutants, with the exception of the most inert chemicals, are likely to undergo complex chemical or photochemical reactions. These can potentially transform a pollutant from its primary physical and chemical state, when entering the atmosphere, to another state that may have similar or very different characteristics. Many volatile organic chemicals (VOCs) e.g., chlorofluorocarbons (CFCs), which have long residence times, are implicated in the depletion of the atmospheric ozone layer. Transformation products may differ from their precursors in chemical stability, toxic properties as well as other characteristics [3-5,7,13].

Atmospheric organic compounds are found in both the gas and particulate phases. The manner in which a given compound partitions will greatly influence that compound's atmospheric removal mechanisms and lifetime, as well as its health effects due to inhalation. The vapour pressure of the compounds, in addition to the amount and type of particulate matter present and temperature, will affect the extent of association with particulate matter. Airborne particulates of respirable size, whether of natural or anthropogenic origin, form an important fraction of all atmospheric aerosols.

Although concentrations of toxic air pollutants near a source may be high, their air concentrations in urban, rural and remote locations can be several orders of magnitude lower than those of ubiquitous type air pollutant. Air concentrations of both vapour and particulate phases tend to decrease rapidly as a function of increasing distance from the emission sources. Atmospheric toxic air pollutants are generally present in the atmosphere at trace concentrations (ppb or ppt), requiring particularly stringent considerations and sophisticated equipment for their collection, separation and quantification [3-5,7,13]. It is also important to distinguish the chemistry of the urban atmosphere considered by Seinfeld [3] to be a "giant reactor in which pollutant gases such as hydrocarbons and oxides of nitrogen and sulphur react under the influence of sunlight to create a variety of products including ozone and submicrometer aerosols" from that of the natural troposphere. While ozone concentrations in unpolluted tropospheric air vary between 20 and 50 ppb, levels as high as 700 ppb have been found in polluted urban areas. The urban atmosphere contains relatively high concentrations of a large number of alkane, alkene, aromatic anthropogenic hydrocarbons compared to the natural troposphere [3].

Natural Sources of Airborne Pollutants

The major *natural* sources of toxic airborne pollutants and some representative examples of toxicant released [13] include:

a)	Crustal rock and soils	Trace and heavy metals (As, Se, Cd, Hg, Pb, Mn)
b)	Volcanic emissions	Heavy metals, sulphur and nitrogen oxides, PAHs
c)	Fires (forest, bush, grass)	PAHs, heavy metals, carbon monoxide, methylchloride
d)	Vegetation and soil erosion	Selenium, zinc, PAHs, methane
e)	Swamps	Hydrogen sulphide, volatile organic compounds

Anthropogenic Sources of Airborne Pollutants

The major *anthropogenic* sources of toxic airborne pollutants and some representative examples of toxicants released [13] include:

a	Industrial processes (manufacturing and commercial operations)	Various organic compounds (e.g. PCBs, industrial solvents); trace metals
b	Pesticide and fertiliser manufacture and use	Chlorinated hydrocarbons nitrogen and phosphorous organic compounds; trace metals
c	Transportation (land, sea, air)	Hydrocarbons and other organic compounds, PAHs, sulphur and nitrogen compounds
d	Waste treatment and disposal	Organic and inorganic compounds, trace metals
e	Combustion process (waste, fossil fuel, biomass)	Heavy metals, trace elements, PAHs, polychlorinated dibenzofurans, methylchloride.

Combustion emission products represent one of the major and most widespread sources of atmospheric pollution. These emissions are very complex mixtures from incomplete burning of materials derived from fossil fuels, vegetative sources or mixtures of these materials (e.g., garbage, waste and coal). The emission mixture consists of gases (e.g., CO, NO_x, SO_2, hydrocarbons and aldehydes), semi-volatile organic compounds (e.g., 2- to 3-ring aromatics), PAHs, polar substituted PAHs and other polar organic compounds, as well as condensed inorganic matter absorbed onto small, usually submicron carbonaceous particles (soot) or non-carbonaceous particles such as silica [10,11,13].

A recent preliminary toxic release chemical inventory compiled by the U.S. Environmental Protection Agency disclosed that some 2.4 billion pounds (approximately 1 billion kg) of toxic air pollutants are released annually into America's air supply. (This figure is based on reports of only 55% to 75% of the total number of companies responding to a questionnaire). Even the total emission figure may be a small percentage of the total since it does not include the thousands of small companies that emit these chemicals but were not included in the inventory). The largest single source of chemical air emissions by more than four-fold is the chemical industry which reported release of some 886.5 million pounds (369 million kg). Other major sources of air emission were primary metals (approximately 90 million kg), paper production (94 million kg), transport equipment (87 million kg) and rubber and plastics production (60 million kg).

Other major contributing industrial sources of the toxic chemical emissions included: fabricated metals, electrical and electronics equipment, petroleum and coals, machinery, furniture and fixtures, instruments, textiles, stone, clay and glass, lumber and food, leather and apparel [16,17]. The above toxic release inventory included more than 320 chemical toxicants (carcinogens, mutagens, neurotoxins and other substances associated with serious human health effects) listed in the Superfund law, a special law adopted in the U.S. on hazardous waste site substances. Sixty of the substances in the inventory are listed as carcinogens by the National Toxicology Programme (NTP) of the U.S. Public Health Service [17]. Releases of listed carcinogens were estimated to be approximately 98 million kg nationally and included (million kg): dichloromethane (methylene chloride) 467.5; benzene, 10.3, chloroform, 9.8, formaldehyde, 6.3, butadiene, 4.1 and carbon tetrachloride, 1.8. Neurotoxins on the list included a number of the most prevalent chemicals in the inventory (million kg): toluene 98.2, xylenes, 50, methylethyl ketone 52, and trichloroethylene, 198.8 [17].

While comparable European estimations are not available, it is at least possible to compare production figures for certain compounds in different parts of the world. The yearly dichloromethane production in the U.S. was 226,000 tons in 1983 and 270,000 tons in Europe in 1980 (WHO, 1988). As about 80% of all dichloromethane produced ends up in the atmosphere, Europe and the U.S. contribute equally to its dispersion in the environment. Worldwide production of benzene is estimated to be about 19 million tons annually, of which about half was produced Europe (WHO, 1988).

For practical purposes, organic air pollutants can be divided into 3 phases according to the different sampling techniques: a) the particulate phase, b) semi-volatile compounds with boiling points higher than 100 °C, and c) the gas phase consisting of smaller and more volatile compounds [18].

Metals and Metalloids

The toxicologically important metals and metalloids such as mercury, cadmium, chromium, nickel, lead, arsenic and selenium are found in significant amounts in the atmosphere as a result of both natural and anthropogenic activities. It is well established that many trace elements are mobilised in association with airborne particles derived from high-temperature combustion sources, e.g., fossil-fuelled power plants, blast furnaces, metallurgical smelters, municipal incinerators and vehicle exhaust [2,6, 19-26].

Combustion of hard coal, lignites and brown coal in electrical power plants and in industrial, commercial and residential burners is the major source of airborne Hg, Mo and Se and a very significant source of As, Cr, Mn, Sb and Tl, while the combustion of oil for the same purpose is the most important source of V and Ni and is an important contributor of Sn. The non-ferrous metal industry accounts for the largest fraction of As, Cd, Cu, Zn and Pb (in addition to petrol combustion) emitted [6].

Chemical, physical and biological effects of airborne metals are a direct function of particle size, concentration and composition. The major parameter governing the significance of natural and anthropogenic emissions of environmentally and toxicologically important metals is particle size. Many elements, notably Pb, Cd, Zn, Cr, V, Ni, Mn and Cu, are found at the highest concentrations in the smallest particles collected from ambient air [20-22].

Stationary sources are the principal contributors of most environmentally and toxically important metals in air. The trend for the immediate future appears to be greater emission of metals (e.g., As, Be, Cd, Cr, Hg, Mn, Ni, Pb, Sb, Se, V and Zn), not only as a result of increased usage patterns but also because of prospective enhanced use of fossil fuels for space heating and electricity generation (whether from conventional coal-fired power plants or new coal technologies such as in-situ gasification, coal pyrolysis, chemical precleaning), particularly in the United States. For example, in 1973, coal use for electrical power generation in the U.S. produced 3.6 million tons of fly ash, 22.6% of the total U.S.

particulate emissions [23]. With the addition of 241 new coal-fired power plants, coal consumption by U.S. electrical utilities expanded from 446 million tons in 1976 to more than 840 million tons and further increasing the amount of fly ash emitted into the atmosphere with concomittant toxic metals.

Global inventories indicate that coal combustion is an important atmospheric source of Hg and As [24,25], while iron and steel production is a significant source of airborne lead. Lead emissions from refuse incineration, although considerable, are small compared with motor vehicle emissions [26].

The major stationary emission sources for Be, Cd, Cr, Mn, Ni, Pb, Ti, and Cu are from smelter metallurgical processing and coal oil combustion. Emissions from incineration are greatly dependent on the composition of the waste material burned [21,27,28]. Many of the metals of higher concentration observed in incinerator atmospheric emissions, e.g., Cr, Pb, Sn, Zn, are metals that are used in surface coatings, galvanising solders and similar surface applications where high temperature could cause flaking and volatilisation from bulk metal scrap [27]. These metals are derived from the combustibles in municipal incinerator emissions.

During incineration, up to 35% of metals in a hazardous waste stream can be emitted into the atmosphere. The stack emissions include As, Cd, Hg, Pb, and Ni [28]. Refuse incineration is a major source of atmospheric cadmium in the United States and United Kingdom [27,29]. The incineration of 3.15 x 10^6 tons/year of refuse in the U.K. has been suggested to yield annual emissions of 6 tons of atmospheric cadmium and 115 tons of atmospheric lead. In the U.S., the incineration of urban refuse may be responsible for major fractions of Zn, Co, Sb and possibly Sn, In, and Ag found in aerosols in many cities [27].

Lantzy and Mackenzie in 1979 [30] presented a comprehensive survey of global data for sources of atmospheric input for 20 trace metals and assessed the relative importance of natural and anthropogenic sources. In addition, a mathematical model was illustrated to calculate enrichment factors which were then compared to the observed factors. The elements considered were: Al, Ti, Sm, Fe, Mn, Co, Cr, V, Ni, Sn, Cu, Cd, Zn, As, Se, Sb, Mo, Ag, Hg, and Pt. The natural emissions included: continental dust flux, volcano dust and gas flux, while the anthropogenic emissions included industrial particulate and fossil fuel emissions. Nriagu [31] described a global inventory of anthropogenic emissions of Cd, Cu, Ni, Pb, and Zn into the atmosphere in 1975. A recent report of Nriagu and Pacryna [6] provides a revision of the earlier data [31] and extends the calculations to many more trace elements.

The following worldwide anthropogenic emissions (median values x 10^3kg/yr) were reported of elements to the atmosphere in 1983 [6]: arsenic: 18,820; cadmium: 7,570; chromium: 30,480; mercury: 3,560; nickel 55,650; lead: 332,350 and selenium: 3,790 (this figure is for particulate Se only, because volatile Se accounts for about 40% of the Se released, the total Se emission was estimated to be 6,320 tons/year). The anthropogenic source categories included: coal and oil combustion (electric utilities, industry and domestic); pyrometallurgical (non-ferrous metal, production, mining, Pb, Cu-Ni and Zn-Cd production); secondary non-ferrous production, steel and iron production, refuse incineration (municipal, sewage waste), phosphate fertilisers, cement production, wood combustion, mobile sources (petrol fuelled). Mean global emissions from natural sources have recently been estimated to be (in tons per year): As 7,800; Cd 1,000; Ni 2,600; Pb 66,000; and Hg 6,000. Approximately 6,000-13,000 times of Se are annually released into the atmosphere from natural sources, with 60-80% of the total Se emission arising from marine biogenic origins. On average, the anthropogenic emission into the atmosphere of As, Cd, Cu, Ni and Zn exceeds the natural inputs of these elements by a factor of 2 or more, while in the case of lead, the ratio of anthropogenic to natural emission rates is about 17 [6].

The impact of acidification (acid rain) on the changing chemical speciation and mobilisation of metals, particularly enhanced for mercury, aluminum, lead and selenium, should be noted.

Arsenic

Apart from arsenic trioxide from volcanic activity, only human activities produce significant air concentrations of this metalloid. Hot metallurgical processes, particularly primary and secondary non-ferrous smelters (e.g., copper, lead, zinc and their alloys), are the major sources of high occupational and local community exposures to arsenic trioxide and cadmium oxide. Large total amounts of both arsenic and cadmium may be released via coal combustion and municipal incinerators. The arsenic concentrations in coal ranges from 0.34 to 130 µg/g and reach 1,500 µg/g in some Czechoslovakian lignites [32]. (Such coals with extensive As levels are used locally and should be considered in estimating the local or even national emission [6].) For example, in Prague, airborne arsenic concentrations were found to be 450 ng/m³ on average in winter and 70 ng/m³ in summer [2]. Additional emissions of arsenic can result from the combustion of wood-containing preservatives, glass enamel making, use of arsenical pesticides, production of high-purity arsenic metal, semiconductor alloys, lead shot and some lead and copper alloys. Soil contamination around industrial sources may be a source of arsenic inhalation exposures (e.g, from soil around smelters contaminated with lead). Trivalent arsenic is oxidised to pentavalent arsenic in the outdoor environment, resulting in some smelter emissions deposited near plant sites having pentavalent arsenic levels. Representative background levels of arsenic (in particulate form as in organic As) in air generally range from 1-10 ng/m³ in rural areas but can reach several hundred ng/m³ in some cities and exceed 1,000 ng/m³ near non-ferrous metal smelters and some power plants, depending on the levels of As in the combusted coal [2].

Cadmium

Cadmium in particulate urban air pollution arises predominantly as the oxide from hot-metal operations and combustion of products containing trace amounts of cadmium (e.g., cadmium pigments, additives to rubber and plastic, metal and sulphate from plating and alloys). Refuse incineration is a major source of atmospheric cadmium release at global level and also in Europe [26]. Other major sources of atmospheric cadmium in Europe

are the steel and zinc production industries [2].

The yearly means of cadmium in air range from <1 to 5 ng/m³ in rural areas, 5-15 ng/m³ in urban areas and 15-50 ng/m³ in industrialised areas. A compilation of Cd levels for Member States of the European Community gave ranges of 0.1-1 ng/m³ for remote areas, 1-50 ng/m³ for urban areas and 1-100 ng/m³ for industrial areas [2].

Some general air pollution (24-hour exposure) levels have been reported for arsenic and cadmium. For arsenic (25-40% deposition and absorption, depending on particle size and chemical form) are 0.02-0.07 µg/m³ or daily pulmonary dose of 0.08-0.28 µg/day. For cadmium (25-90% deposition and absorption, depending on compound and particle size distribution), 0.002-0.05 µg/m³ or daily pulmonary dose 0.008-0.2 µg/day [33].

Mercury

Mercury is emitted into the atmosphere via various natural and anthropogenic sources. The natural sources include: volcanoes, soil erosion, wind-blown dust, crystal degassing, geysers and forest firs. The human sources of atmospheric mercury include chlor-alkali plants, cement manufacturing, mining, smelting and refining of ores, combustion of fossil fuels and biomass, waste disposal and paint production and use [2,6,34].

On a global basis, current anthropogenic emissions of mercury into the troposphere are estimated to be of similar order of magnitude as pre-industrial emissions from natural sources. It is expected that increased fossil fuel consumption for industrial, commercial or domestic purposes will further increase the anthropogenic contribution of atmospheric mercury [34]. In Europe, anthropogenic emissions of mercury in 1985 were expected to total 2,630 tons, of which 765 tons would be emitted into the atmosphere while total natural emissions would amount to 570 tons, nearly all (527 tons) being emitted into the atmosphere [2].

Emission measurements and mass balance calculations performed at coal-burning power stations suggest that 80-100% of the mercury in coal escapes into the atmosphere as elemental mercury vapour rather than in particulate form. Metallic mercury appears to be highly anomalous existing in ambient air, primarily as the reduced elemental form since the atmosphere possesses well-known oxidising capacity (e.g., photochemical smog and oxidation of acid rain precursors such as SO_2 and NO_2). Additionally, most metals exist in ambient air as oxides or other compounds with chemical oxidation states greater than zero (e.g., metal sulphates, nitrates or chlorides).

Elemental mercury vapour has an estimated residence time in the atmosphere of at least several months and perhaps even 1 or 2 years, in contrast to mercury associated with particulate matter which would be expected to have an atmospheric residence time of only a few weeks or less. However, it is still broadly acknowledged that much unambiguous information remains to be known concerning the chemical forms, transformations and lifetimes of mercury species in the atmosphere. For example, it has been postulated that since there is a widespread presence in the troposphere of oxidants such as OH radicals, H_2O_2, ozone and various oxygenated organic species, mercury (II) oxide is likely to be one of a number of inorganic mercury compounds in the atmosphere. Additionally, conditions for the formation of HgO also exist in plumes from fossil fuel power-generating plants and probably other stationary or mobile sources as well.

Background levels of mercury in the troposphere of the Northern hemisphere are estimated at 2 ng/m^3. In areas of Europe remote from industrial activity, mean concentrations of total mercury in the atmosphere are normally in the range of 2-3 ng/m^3 in the summer and 3-4 ng/m^3 in the winter [2]. Concentrations of atmospheric mercury reported in Member States of the European Community range from 0.001-6 ng/m^3 in remote areas, 0.1-5 ng/m^3 in urban areas to 0.5 - 20 ng/m^3 in industrial areas [2,35].

Lead Compounds

A variety of alkyl lead species may be present in the environment as a result of tetra-alkyl lead emissions from motor vehicles and the environmental decomposition of these compounds [36]. The presence of tetra-alkyl lead compounds in air has been known for some time. These compounds are used as petrol additives and their potential sources associated with this use are evaporation at petrol stations, spillages and effluents from tetraalkyl lead manufacture. Recently, the occurrence of gas phase trialkyl lead and dialkyl lead species has been demonstrated [37]. In the atmosphere, tetraaklyl lead compounds decompose to trialkyl lead, dialkyl lead and inorganic Pb^{+2} principally via reaction with OH radicals. Half-lives of 5-10 hours for tetramethyl lead and 0-2 hours for tetraethyl lead were estimated for the summer months. Trialkyl lead species also react with OH radical but the reaction rates are slower than for tetraalkyl lead compounds. Half-lives of 5 days for trimethyl lead were evaluated, suggesting that trialkyl lead compounds are fairly persistent intermediates in the atmospheric decomposition of tetraalkyl lead. Reported concentrations of vapour phase alkyl lead compounds have also been measured in atmospheric particules at concentrations of the order of picograms Pb/m^3, suggesting that this is not a significant component in comparison to vapour phase alkyl lead [36].

Most of the lead in the air is in the form of fine particles with a mass median equivalent diameter of 1 micron. The organic level fraction (principally lead alkyls) that escaped combustion is generally below 10% of the total atmospheric lead, with over 90% of lead from leaded petrol emitted as inorganic particles, e.g., PbBrCl [2]. Atmospheric concentrations of lead range from 0.0001-0.001 μg/m^3 in areas remote from civilisation. It has been estimated from geochemical data that the concentration of lead of natural origin in air is about 0.0006 μg/m^3 [38]. Natural concentrations result from airborne dust, containing on the average 10-15 μg/g lead, and from gases diffusing from the earth's crust [39,40]. Current "baseline" levels of lead in the atmosphere are estimated to be in the range of 5 x 10^{-5} ug/m^3 [2,41]. In rural areas, levels of lead range from 0.1 to 0.3 μg/m^3, while in non-urban sites located near urban sites air lead averages about 0.5 μg/m^3. Higher concentrations of lead in ambient air are found in urban areas with high traffic density. Currently, in most European cities, urban air lead levels are in the range of 0.5 to 3.0 ug/m^3 (annual means) [2]. Analysis of air samples collected in the US between 1965 and 1974 from 92 urban and 16 non-urban sites showed that composite lead concentrations in air were highest (1.1 µg/m³) in 1971 but had declined to 0.84 µg/m³ by 1973 [40]. With the lowering of the lead content in petrol (and eventual elimination), there is a trend toward lower air lead values in the the U.S. and certain areas of Europe [2,40].

Chromium

Chromium in air can arise from both natural sources (e.g., wind erosion of shales, clays and many kinds of soil containing chromium) as well as from anthropogenic sources including chromite mining, metallurgical processes, the combustion of coal, cement-producing plants, wearing of brake linings, catalytic emission and control systems in vehicles [2,40,42].

During the period of 1960-1969, approximately 200 urban stations in the U.S. had annual mean concentrations of 0.1-0.03 µg/m³ chromium, while in non-urban areas the level is less than 0.01 µg/m³ [40].

In many urban and rural areas of the U.S., the chromium concentrations were in the range of 5.2 ng/m³ (24-hour background level) to 156.8 ng/m³; (urban annual average) during the period 1977-1980 [2,43]. In a recent survey, ranges of chromium levels in Member States of the European Community were reported as following: remote areas 0-3 ng/m³; urban areas 4-70 ng/m³; and industrial areas 5-200 ng/m³ [2,35]. In addition, chromium ranges in air of 1-140 ng/m³ in continental Europe, 45-67 ng/m³ in Hawaii and 20-70 ng/m³ in Japan have also been reported [2,44]. Mass median diameters of chromium particles in the ambient air have been reported to be in the range of 1.5-1.9 microns [2,35].

Nickel

The major anthropogenic sources of nickel emissions to the atmosphere include the combustion of coal, residual and fuel oils and municipal waste and nickel mining and refining [2]. Coal and oil combustion are the prin-

cipal sources of nickel emission in the U.S., with the combustion of oil accounting for 60-98% of the nickel emitted [2,45]. Nickel-containing particles released from oil combustion in the California urban area were in the fine-size fractions below 1 micron, while in coal-fired plants nickel enrichment occured in the smaller particulate fraction (<1 micron) [2,22]. Nickel sulphate is the major nickel species in air [2]. The total annual nickel global emissions from anthropogenic sources has been reported to range from 4.3×10^{10} - 9.8×10^{10} compared to 3×10^{10} - 0.85×10^{10} from natural sources (volcanic gases and dusts, continental dusts) [2,30,46]. Average particulate concentrations form nickel have been reported to range from 0-0.6 ng/m³ in remote areas, 9-50 ng/m³ in semiremote areas and 60-300 ng/m³ in urban locations [2]. Nickel concentration ranges for Member States of the European Community were 0.1-0.7 ng/m³ in remote areas, 3-100 ng/m³ in urban and 8-200 ng/m³ in industrial areas [2,35]. The daily dustfall deposition rates in this survey were: 0.20-10 µg/m² in remote areas, 2-10 µg/m³ in urban areas and 7-70 µg/m² in industrialised areas [2,35]. Nickel concentrations of particulate matter as high as 3,310 µg/m³ have been found in the ambient air of nickel-processing centres [2]. Particle size measurements of nickel in both urban and remote areas showed mass median aerodynamic diameters of 0.83 - 1.67 µm (US urban), 1.2 µm (Toronto urban), 0.6 µm (England, rural). At least 50% of airborne nickel is in particles of <2-3 µm diameter [2,47].

Polynuclear Aromatic Hydrocarbons (PAHs)

Polynuclear aromatic hydrocarbons (PAHs) are formed by the incomplete combustion of almost any fuel, (e.g., fossil, biomass, wood) and are transported through the atmosphere in the vapour phase and absorbed on particulate matter [2,18,48-51]. Thus the urban atmosphere environment contains many organic trace pollutants (primarily PAHs and long-chain aliphatic hydrocarbons) that are related to incomplete fuel combustion in domestic heating, industrial plants and vehicular traffice. In ambient aerosol these compounds will distribute between the gas phase and aerosol.

The ratio of PAHs in the vapour and particulate phase of urban and rural samples in ambient air vary considerably with the season and the scavenging effect of snow and rain [18]. The daytime decay of PAHs on atmospheric soot particles has been shown to be influenced by humidity, sunlight and temperature. Although 500 PAHs have been detected in air, most measurements have been made on benzo(a)pyrene (BaP) [2,50,52].

It should be noted that data reported on atmospheric levels of the PAHs prior to the mid 1970s may be comparable only to a limited extent with later data, due to different sampling and analytical procedures [2]. The relation between the level of BaP and some other PAHs is termed the "PAH profile" and if PAH profiles are determined by a routine method, only 6-15 of the several hundred existing PAHs are measured quantitatively [2].

The total annual release of PAHs from mobile sources in the United States has been estimated. In the case of benzo(a)pyrene, all mobile sources produced about 43 tons in 1979, including 27 tons from motor vehicles; 63% and 37% of the BaP emission from motor vehicles occurred in urban and rural areas, respectively. It was projected that the total motor vehicle BaP emission in the U.S. will decrease by the year 2000 to 24 tons, of which only about 40% will be in urban areas [49]. On the basis of motor vehicle emission values for 1979, the average daily BaP concentration in the urban atmosphere in the U.S. was calculated as 1.3 ng/m^3 (49). United States annual BaP atmospheric emission from all combustion sources, including both mobile and stationary sources, was estimated at between 300 and 1,300 tons [49].

The emissions into the air of benzo(a)pyrene from several sources in the Federal Republic of Germany in 1981 were estimated to amount to 18 tons, of which 56% was caused by heating with coal, 30% by coal production, 13% by motor vehicles and less than 0.5% by heating with oil and coal-fired power generation [2,52] (Earlier BaP emissions resulting from the use of hard-coal briquettes for heating purposes was much higher since such briquettes were made employing a binder with 7% pitch which contained 1% BaP [2].)

The natural background level of BaP in air (excluding forest fires) may be nearly zero. In the 1970s, the annual average of BaP in urban areas without coal-ovens in the U.S. was less than 1 ng/m^3 and other cities between 1 and 5 ng/m^3.

In a number of European cities in the 1960s the annual average concentration of BaP was higher than 100 ng/m^3, but in the Federal Republic of Germany and the United Kingdom the concentrations of BaP have fallen dramatically in recent decades due to controls on smoke emissions and the virtual disappearance of the open coal fire for domestic heating purposes [2]. However, coal burning in small domestic open fires or stoves produces levels of BaP that are several magnitudes higher than those emitted by oil-fuel central heating systems [2,52]. Additionally, some areas near industrial sources can have relatively high levels of BaP in the ambient air (e.g., levels of 40 ng BaP/m^3) have been found near coke-oven plants [2].

Many uncertainties remain regarding the persistence of PAHs, their chemical transformation and their transport and fate in the atmosphere [48,49]. For example, there are reports that PAHs degrade quickly in the atmosphere with a lifetime as short as several hours. In contrast, a number of reports suggest that PAHs degrade slowly, if at all, in the atmosphere and eventually deposit on soil or water. This is supported by studies of marine sediments, the ultimate environmental sinks of PAHs. These studies have shown that the relative abundance of PAHs, even at the most remote locations, are similar to those in combustion sources, suggesting that PAHs are stable in the atmosphere.

There is increasing evidence that a number of PAHs can react with atmospheric oxidants, (e.g., peroxyacetyl nitrate (PAN), nitric and nitrous acid) to form various nitroarenes whose toxicity (primarily mutagenicity) is often greater than that of the parent compound [53]. Pitts [53] demonstrated that gas-phase reaction of several PAHs abundant in urban atmosphere react with OH radical in the presence of NO_x during the day time, and with N_2O_5 at night to produce nitroarenes, (e.g., 2-NO_2-fluoranthene, 1-NO_2-pyrene, 2-NO_2-pyrene). It should also be noted that a number of nitroarenes have been found in primary emissions of diesel soot (e.g., 1-NO_2-pyrene, 3-NO_2-fluoranthene and 8-NO_2-fluoranthene) [53-55].

Arey et al. [56] reported that in ambient atmospheres the nitro-derivatives of the 2-ring PAH may be significantly more abundant than the particle-associated nitrofluoranthenes and nitropyrenes. It was shown that the majority of nitroarenes present in the ambient air are formed from the gas-phase reactions of N_2O_5 and/or the OH radical in the presence of NO_x.

Photochemical Oxidants

It is well recognised that photochemical oxidants present in polluted air can significantly impair human lung function.

Peroxyacyl nitrates (PANs)

Peroxyacyl nitrate (PAN), which is the most abundant of the PANs, is formed by the photochemical reactions of acetaldehyde in the presence of NO_2. Peroxyacyl nitrates are an important reservoir for NO_x in the atmosphere [2-5,57].

Other aldehydes present in the atmosphere may also react to form PANs. For example, peroxypropionyl nitrate, peroxylbutyryl nitrate and peroxybenzyl nitrate are all produced by analogous reactions of the respective aldehyde (e.g., propionaldehyde, butyraldehyde and benzaldehyde, respectively) [58].

It has also been suggested that, in the atmosphere, peroxyglutaryl nitrate (PGN) may be formed by the reaction of OH with the dialdehyde glutaraldehyde in the presence of NO_2.

Glutaraldehyde is one of the most abundant dialdehydes in urban atmosphere found at concentrations up to 0.3 $\mu g/m^3$ (0.1 ppb), and is a product of the photochemical degradation of cyclopentene [59].

Peroxyacetyl nitrate concentrations have been reported to reach maximum values of 80 $\mu g/m^3$ in the U.S. and 90 $\mu g/m^3$ in the Netherlands; in the latter country an increase in this oxidant's concentrations has been noted in the last decade [2].

Hydrogen peroxide

Hydrogen peroxide is produced in the atmosphere through a series of photochemical reactions involving anthropogenic hydrocarbons and NO_x trace gases [60]. Recent measurements have shown that H_2O_2 is present over the Northeast United States at concentrations up to 4 ppb (v) in autumn, approximately one-tenth of typical ozone concentrations. Other calculations of H_2O_2 atmospheric concentrations in other regions are in the range of 1 ppb to about 50 ppb, with an uncertainty of about one order of magnitude depending on the data input used in modelling [61]. Hydrogen peroxide is a strong oxidant and has been suggested to be involved in the formation of H_2SO_4 and HNO_3 and of the corresponding salts from the respective precursors SO_2 and NO_x.

Ozone - Natural and Anthropogenic Sources

Ozone is an allotrope of oxygen that occurs naturally in the planetary boundary layer. It has been implicated, to varying degrees and under specified atmospheric conditions, to the chemical and physical processes in ambient air that produce such particulate and aerosol-related phenomena as acid precipitation and deposition, atmospheric visibility reduction and climate modification [2-5]. Ozone is a highly reactive gas and a strong oxidant and reacts rapidly and selectively with many organic compounds. Ozone is also produced in the atmosphere through a series of photochemical reactions involving anthropogenic hydrocarbons and NO_x trace gases [2-5,60].

Ozone is formed when ultraviolet radiation dissociates molecular oxygen at high altitudes (above 20 km):

$$O_2 + uv \rightarrow 2O \qquad (a)$$
$$O + O_2 + M \rightarrow O_3 + M \qquad (b)$$

where M represents another molecule of oxygen or nitrogen that is unchanged in the reaction [3,4]. At lower altitudes, where only radiation with wavelengths greater than 280 nm is present, the only significant oxygen atom production is from photo-dissociation of nitrogen dioxide:

$$NO_2 + uv \rightarrow NO + O \qquad (c)$$

The nitric oxide produced in this reaction reacts rapidly with ozone to regenerate NO_2:

$$NO + O_3 \rightarrow NO_2 + O_2 \qquad (d)$$

Reactions (b-d) occur rapidly establishing a steady state ozone concentration [3,4]. In its steady state, the ozone concentration can be described as:

$$O_3 \text{ concentration} = \frac{\text{Constant} \times NO_2 \text{ concentration}}{NO \text{ concentration}}$$

The maximum ozone concentration that can be reached in polluted atmospheres appears to depend not only on the absolute concentrations of volatile organic compounds and nitrogen dioxides but also on their ratio [2]. Conditions are favourable for the formation of appreciable levels of ozone at intermediate rations of 4:1 to 10:1 [2]. There are no significant anthropogenic emissions of ozone into the atmosphere [2].

The primary source of excess tropospheric ozone is the reaction between hydrocarbons and oxides of nitrogen emitted from the combustion of fossil fuels [2-5,60,61].

With respect to source emission of ozone, there remains substantial uncertainty concerning the effect of naturally occurring (biogenic) organic precursor emissions on rural ozone concentrations [64]. Biogenic organic species, mostly isoprene and several monoterpenes, are emitted by many types of forest trees and cultivated plants. There are seasonal and geographical differences between the biogenic organic emission rates. Isoprene can contribute as much as 50% of the overall reactivity of rural air, even though its concentration is as low as 6% of the ambient hydrocarbon level [63]. These species (isoprene and monoterpenes) are rapidly oxidised into a number of intermediate species such as methyl vinyl ketone, methyl glyoxal and formaldehyde, which are also highly reactive.

The atmosphere concentration of ozone ranges from 0.02-10 ppm (volume), with an atmospheric lifetime of less than a few hours. However, the lifetime of O_x (ozone and oxygen atoms) depends strongly on location, varying from about an hour in the upper stratosphere to months in the lower stratosphere to hours to days in the troposphere [2-5,60,61]. Seasonal variations in ozone concentration occur which are caused principally by changes in meterological processes, while diurnal patterns of ozone vary according to location, depending on the balance of factors affecting ozone formation, transport and decomposition [2,5]. Long-range transport of ozone and/or its precursors from upwind source areas or from a tropospheric origin is responsible where elevated ozone concentrations have been measured in rural areas having insignificant local sources of ozone precursors [2]. Long-range transport of ozone between urban areas has become increasingly evident [64]. Maximum hourly ozone concentrations exceeding 200 $\mu g/m^3$ have been found in rural areas of Norway and Sweden and 300 $\mu g/m^3$ in rural areas of the U.S [2]. Maximum hourly ozone values of 380 and 520 $\mu g/m^3$ have been measured in the Netherlands and U.K [2]. In the U.S., 1-hour mean concentrations of ozone often exceed 400 $\mu g/m^3$ [2,65] and in certain parts of Europe, urban 1-hour mean ozone concentrations exceed 350 $\mu g/m^3$ [2]. Principally as a result of scavenging of ozone by nitric oxide originating in traffic, ozone concentrations in city centres are often lower than those in the suburbs [2].

Ozone Depletion Precursors: Chloroflurocarbons (CFCs) and Halocarbons

Although the CFCs were first discovered in 1930 and the demand for these agents grew dramatically from 1946 through the mid 1970s, due to their broad utility as aerosol propellants, blowing agents, refrigerants and for air conditioning, it was only relatively recently that the danger they pose was recognised. A steady stream of scientific evidence linking the erosion of the stratosphere ozone layer to chlorine compounds has been accumulating since 1974, when Rowland and

Molina first predicted that the CFCs would cause a very slow loss of stratospheric ozone over the entire globe, thereby exposing humans, animals and plant life to harmful levels of ultraviolet radiation. The recent discovery of a stratospheric ozone hole (resulting in sudden drop of 50% of Antartic ozone concentration), believed to be principally caused by the release of CFCs into the atmosphere and the subsequent formation of chlorine monoxide, has hightened the concern. Although most degradation of ozone by the CFCs occurs in the lower atmosphere, the CFCs contribute some chlorine to the stratosphere [3-5,66].

A variety of mechanisms have been suggested to account for the destruction of ozone [3-5]. Free atomic chlorine is produced by the photodissociation of compounds with long atmospheric lifetimes such as the chlorofluorocarbons:

$$CCl_2F_2 + uv \longrightarrow CClF_2 + Cl$$
$$CCl_3F + uv \longrightarrow CCl_2 + Cl$$

The odd nitrogen and hydrogen radicals and atomic chlorine participate in catalytic cycles that destroy the ozone such as the following:

$$Cl + O_3 \longrightarrow ClO + O_2 \qquad (1)$$
$$ClO + O \longrightarrow Cl + O_2$$
$$\overline{\rule{0pt}{0pt}\hspace{5cm}}$$
$$O_3 + O \longrightarrow 2O_2 \text{ (net)}$$

$$NO + O_3 \longrightarrow NO + O_2 \qquad (2)$$
$$NO_2 + O \longrightarrow NO + O_2$$
$$\overline{\rule{0pt}{0pt}\hspace{5cm}}$$
$$O_3 + O \longrightarrow 2O_2 \text{ (net)}$$

$$OH + O_3 \longrightarrow HO_2 + O_2 \qquad (3)$$
$$HO_2 + O \longrightarrow OH + O_2$$
$$\overline{\rule{0pt}{0pt}\hspace{5cm}}$$
$$O_3 + O \longrightarrow 2O_2 \text{ (net)}$$

Since the atomic oxygen that reacts in the second reaction in each of the above cycles otherwise would have formed ozone, the net effect of each cycle is the destruction of 2 ozone molecules [4].

Most of the world's CFCs are produced and consumed in developed countries in the Northern hemisphere. The depletion of the ozone belt could be most severe at latitudes above 40° in the Northern and Southern hemispheres. Affected would be the northern part of the United States, Canada, most of Europe, the USSR and parts of the Peoples Republic of China, according to one projection [67]. For the period 1978 to 1984 the ozone layer eroded at an annual rate of 0.5% [67]. CFCs not only catalyse destruction of ozone in the upper atmosphere, but are themselves greenhouse gases like carbon dioxide and absorb and re-radiate back towards the earth's surface some of the infrared radiation that would escape to space. Concentrations of CFCs and halocarbons are rising faster than those of most greenhouse gases because their annual rate of release has been increasing in recent years. The concentrations of $CFCl_3$ (CFC-11), which was used as an aerosol propellant and is still employed as a blowing agent for foam insulation, and CF_2Cl_2 (CFC-12), a refrigerant, are growing about 5% annually while the concentration of $CCl_2FCCl_2F_2$ (CFC-113), a solvent for cleaning electronic microcircuits, is soaring at an annual rate of 11% [62]. The United States, European Community and Australia consume most CFCs, with an estimated per capita consumption in the U.S. alone of approximately 0.82 kg of CFC-11 and CFC-12, compared to Japanese consumption of approximately 0.5 kg per capita of CFC-11 and CFC-12 [67].

The atmospheric concentration of $CFCl_3$ (CFC-11) is 2.3×10^{-4} ppm (volume) with an atmospheric lifetime of 75 years, while CF_2Cl_2 (CFC-12) is found at an atmospheric concentration of 3×10^{-4} ppm (volume) with an atmospheric lifetime of 110 years [62].

Recently, steps have been taken on an international level to abate the ozone depletion crisis. Thirty-six nations have ratified the Montreal Protocol which went into effect January 1, 1989, requiring that production of CFCs be reduced to 50% of 1986 levels by mid-1998, and Halon production be frozen in 1992 at 1986 levels. In August 1988, the U.S. Environmental Protection Agency issued regulations to implement the terms domestically.

The atmospheric levels of several other important halocarbons are increasing rapidly. These include carbon tetrachloride, which is used in the production of CFC-11 and CFC-12, methyl chloroform, which is used as a solvent for cleaning sheet metal and is a cleaning agent in the electronics industry, and the fire retardants CF_3Br (Halon 1301) and CF_2BRCl (Halon 1211).

Methyl chloroform has a much shorter lifetime (about 6.5 years) than the fully halogenated gases. Although halocarbons that have hydrogen atoms can be consumed in the troposphere by hydroxyl radicals, there are currently 130 ppt of methyl chloroform in the atmosphere and it is increasing at a rate of about 7% per year. Carbon tetrachloride, with a lifetime of about 50 years, has an atmospheric concentration of about 125 ppt that is growing at an annual rate of about 1% [4]. These gases contribute to the destruction of ozone and to greenhouse warming [62]. The CFCs are believed to contribute approximately 17% to global warming [68].

Even with the projected phaseout of the CFCs by the late 1990s, the stratospheric concentrations of chlorine will continue to grow. By the year 2010, chlorine concentrations are projected to be about 3 times as large as the current level of about 3 ppt, largely due to the projected increase in the use of carbon tetrachloride and methyl chloroform [66].

Hydrocarbons

A large number of hydrocarbons (e.g., saturated and unsaturated aliphatic, aromatic, polycyclic and halogenated hydrocarbons) have been found in the atmosphere [1,69]. For example, more than 130 alkanes have been identified; of those detected in ambient air, about two-thirds are found in the gas phase and about one-third in the aerosol phase. A large number have been found indoors and the higher alkanes are found in rain and snow as well [69]. Nearly 150 alkenes and alkynes have been found in the gas phase, being somewhat more common than in the aerosol phase. By far the largest source of alkanes, alkenes and alkynes is the combustion of fossil fuels. Nearly a hundred monocyclic hydrocarbons have been detected, about two-thirds in the gas phase with the great majority arising from the combustion of fossil fuel or biomass. More than 70 aromatic hydrocarbons (e.g., benzene and its derivatives) have been found in the atmosphere, most often in the gas phase, and are produced by fossil fuel combustion and a broad variety of industrial processes [69].

Methane

Levels of methane, one of the fastest growing of greenhouse gases, have risen dramatically in recent years. Each year an additional 50 million tons of methane remain in the air, producing the current concentration (about 1.7 ppm), which is estimated to be more than twice as high as it was before the industrial revolution. Since systematic measurements of atmospheric methane began in 1979, levels of methane have grown more than 1% annually [62]. More than half of the methane released into the atmosphere originates from the action of anaerobic bacteria on plant material, in rice paddies and wetlands of all types in all latitudes and the stomachs of ruminants such as cattle and sheep. Methane is also emitted from the incomplete combustion of vegetation in forest or range fires or when land is cleared for agriculture. Additionally, methane is released from coal mines, leaks in natural gas pipelines, leaks of natural gas associated with oil production and decomposition of organic matter in landfills [62].

Methane has a lifetime of about 9 years due to its oxidation with hydroxyl radical in the troposphere. Residual quantities of tropospheric methane escape to the stratosphere, where it is destroyed [62].

Ethylene and Propylene

Ethylene is extensively employed in a broad spectrum of chemical and polymer production and some dissipative losses could be expected to occur. Ethylene is produced by all plant tissues, by soil micro-organisms including fungi and bacteria and has also been detected in marsh gas and gases desorbed from coal samples [70]. In the U.S., ethylene concentrations in the air varied from 29-88 $\mu g/m^3$ [25-77 ppb] in downtown Los Angeles, from 21-24 $\mu g/m^3$ (18-21 ppb) in Auzua, California, from 805 $\mu g/m^3$ (700 ppb) in the centre of Washington, D.C. to 45 $\mu g/m^3$ (39 ppb) in an outlying suburb and from 7 $\mu g/m^3$ (6.1 ppb) to 8.2 mg/m^3 (7100 ppb) in the Houston, Texas area [70]. Ethylene concentrations in the air of rural areas in the UK varied over a 2-year period from 0.53-11.5 $\mu g/m^3$ (0.46-10 ppb) with a mean of 2.64 $\mu g/m^3$ (2.3 ppb). Ethylene concentrations in the air near Delft, the Netherlands, average 18 $\mu g/m^3$ (15.5 ppb) [70].

Propylene is extensively employed in chemical synthesis and polymer production, principally in the production of polypropylene, acrylonitrile, isopropyl alcohol and propylene oxide (FO). It has been detected in urban air at levels of 1-10 $\mu g/m^3$ and rural air at levels of 0.10-8.2 $\mu g/m^3$ [70]. Propylene has been found in vehicle exhausts [70].

Butadiene

1,3-Butadiene is a major industrial commodity in the U.S., western Europe and Japan, with broad utility in polymer production. It has been detected in urban air in the U.S. at an average concentration of 0.002 $\mu g/m^3$. Levels of 1,3-butadiene of 0.004 $\mu g/m^3$ in Denver, CO; <0.001-0.028 mg/m^3 in the various Texas cities, and levels as high as 0.02 mg/m^3 in urban air in the Los Angeles/Riverside, California area have all been reported [71]. In the U.S., combined levels of 1,3-butadiene and 2-butene of 5.9-24.4 ppb (0.01-0.05 mg/m^3) in Tulsa, Oklahoma and 0-0.042 mg/m^3) in Houston, Texas have also been reported [71]. Butadiene has been found in cigarette smoke and vehicle exhausts.

Benzene

Benzene is a major industrial chemical produced in enormous quantities which has extensive utility in the production of a large number of substituted aromatic hydrocarbons. U.S. petrols contain an average of 0.8% benzene and European petrols an average of 5%, with occasional levels reaching 16% [2,72]. The total global annual cycle, including benzene in fossil fuels, is estimated to be 32 million tons, of which 4 million tons are believed to be lost to the environment [73]. The major sources of emission of benzene are from motor vehicles and evaporation losses during the handling, distribution and storage of petrol [2,73]. Benzene comprises

about 2.15% of total hydrocarbon emission from a petrol engine or about 4% of automotive exhaust [73,74]. Benzene emitted into the atmosphere has a half-life of less than one day [2,75]. Benzene concentrations in ambient air are generally between 3 and 160 $\mu g/m^3$ (0.001-0.05 ppm) and higher ambient benzene levels are found in metropolitan areas [2,72,74]. In the vicinity of petrol stations and storage tanks and benzene-producing/handling industries, concentrations of benzene at levels of up to several hundred $\mu g/m^3$ have been reported [2,72,74].

Methyl Chloride

Methyl chloride, widely employed in the production of alkyl lead anti-knock agents and methyl silicone polymers and resins, is the most abundant of the nearly 70 alkanic halogenated derivatives found in the troposphere. Its emission occurs from both natural and anthropogenic sources [69,76]. The average global atmospheric concentration is estimated to be in the order of 1 ppb (2.1 $\mu g/m^3$) with the lower concentrations (0.6-0.8 ppb) (1.2-1.7 $\mu g/m^3$) in rural areas and higher concentrations in urban areas and near localised sources [76]. The principal sources of methyl chloride are formed in the oceans by seaweeds and marine micro-organisms and by the various combustion processes of organic matter (e.g., forest fires, slash-and-burn agriculture, fossil fuels, incineration of domestic, municipal and industrial rubbish, accidental fires and cigarettes) [76,77]. The major source of atmospheric methyl chloride is the oceans which release 1,000-8,000 million kg/year; urban sources and the combustion of vegetation are estimated to release 150-600 million kg/year while emission from the manufacture, processing and distribution of methyl chloride contributed about 20 million kg in 1980 [76,77].

The primary mechanism for the removal of atmospheric methylchloride is believed to be reaction with hydroxyl radicals. The residence time of methyl chloride in an urban atmosphere is estimated to be 231 days with a daily rate loss (12 sunlit hours) of 0.4% [76]. Average levels of methyl chloride in air at 10 urban sites in the U.S. ranged form 0.7-3.0 ppb (1.4-6.2 $\mu g/m^3$) and the calculated average human exposures to methyl chloride at these sites ranged up to 140 µg/person/day [76-79]. Measurements of methyl chloride in the air of Southern England between December 1974 and April 1975 showed a mean concentration of 1.1 ppb (2.3 µg/m^3) while the average concentration in the stratosphere over France in 1978 was calculated to be approximately 0.7 ppb (1.5 µg/m^3) [76].

Nitrogen Oxides (NO$_X$)

Although many chemical species of nitrogen oxides exist, nitrogen dioxide is the predominant form from the point of atmospheric significance on local, regional and global scales as well as for human health [2-5]. In the lower atmosphere, NO$_x$ is involved in the photochemical production of ozone and with sulphur oxides (SO$_x$), which contribute to acidic wet and dry deposition [3-5,14]. The major source of emissions of NO$_x$ into the atmosphere is the combustion of fossil fuels in stationary sources (heating and power generation) and internal combustion engines in motor vehicles. The nitrogen oxides that are emitted in the flue gas of power plants consist of about 95% nitric oxide (NO) and 5% NO$_2$. After emission, NO is converted to NO$_2$ via oxidation with atmospheric ozone [2-5,80]. The oxidation rate of NO depends on a number of important factors, including the molecular reaction rates and physical kinetics (the processes of dispersion and mixing of the plume with ambient air). Chemical and physical kinetics depend on meteorological conditions such as wind speed and solar radiation and on concentration of the reactants [80]. Nitrogen-containing air pollutants such as HNO$_3$, aerosol nitrates and peroxyacyl nitrate (PAN), are formed as further reaction products of NO$_2$ in the atmosphere. For NO$_x$, the largest source of anthropogenic emissions excluding combustion of fossil fuels is the burning of biomass. Other contributions of NO$_x$ to the atmosphere arise from the manufacture of nitric acid and the use of explosives and welding processes [2]. Differences in NO$_x$ emissions of various countries can be attributed principally to differences in fossil fuel combustion. Global emissions of NOx in 1970 were estimated at approximately 53 million tons [2,81]. Annual mean NO$_2$ con-

centrations in urban areas throughout the world are generally in the range of 20-90 µg/m^3 (0.01-0.05 ppm) [2]. Urban outdoor levels of NO$_2$ vary according to seasonal, diurnal and meteorological factors with typically higher levels from peak traffic emissions of NO [2-5]. The maximal hourly mean value of NO$_2$ may be 3-10 times the annual mean [2]. Monitoring activities over the last 2 decades indicate an increase in NO$_x$ in urban areas throughout the world [2-5,85]. Changes in combustion-generated emission of NO$_x$ (and SO$_x$) between 1966 and 1980 show that NO$_x$ and SO$_x$ are very unevenly distributed globally, resulting in large local and regional variations from the global mean fluxes. The greatest rates of emission of NO$_x$ and SO$_x$ from fossil-fuel combustion between 1966 and 1980 occurred in the northern mid-latitudes, while the greatest increases during this period have taken place in the tropics [79]. Emissions of NO$_X$ in the U.S. in 1985 were stated to be 20.6 million tons [82]. Nitrogen oxides are widely found in indoor air.

Nitrous Oxide

Nitrous oxide (N$_2$O) emissions into the atmosphere are considered to arise primarily from anthropogenic sources, e.g., large stationary combustion sources. For combustion systems fired with coal or heavy oil, measured N$_2$O emissions averaged 25% of the total NO$_x$ concentration. Emissions at this level are suggested to explain the observed increase in atmospheric N$_2$O (e.g., an annual rate of 0.18-0.26%), although it has been suggested that denitrification of chemical fertilisers and biomass burning could account for the observed increase in atmospheric N$_2$O. Nitrous oxide, whose average tropospheric lifetime is 150 years, contributes to greenhouse warming and supply of nitrous oxide to the stratosphere, where it destroys ozone. The only known atmospheric sink for nitrous oxide is its breakdown to nitric oxide in the stratosphere by ultraviolet light. Concentrations of nitrous oxide are climbing steadily, rising from 280 ppb at the turn of the century to about 300 ppb at present (which is one-thousandth of CO$_2$ concentrations). This results from the injection of 5 million tons of N$_2$O into the atmosphere each year. It has been suggested that doubling of the present N_2O concentration would effect a 12% decrease in total ozone.

Sulphur Oxides (SOx)

Sulphur oxides (sulphur dioxide, acid aerosols resulting from the oxidation of SO_2 in the atmosphere and SO_2 plus particulate matter), primarily derived from the combustion of fossil fuels, are major air pollutants in urban areas of the world [2-5,7-16,82,84]. In addition, there are some natural sources of SO_2, such as volcanoes, that also contribute to environmental levels in the European region and elsewhere [2].

Declining use in the types or amounts of fossil fuel used during the last 2 decades has resulted in declining emissions of SO_x in the U.S. and certain areas of Europe. Nevertheless, Europe and the U.S. each emit about 25 million tons more of SO_2 than Africa [85]. Additionally, the change from multiple domestic, commercial or industrial sources towards large single sources (power stations) that disperse pollutants at higher altitudes, has led to significant reductions in concentrations of SO_x in many previously highly polluted large cities [2,4,5]. However, this has resulted in a more widespread distribution via long-distance transport in Europe and elsewhere [2]. The annual mean levels of SO_2 in major cities of Europe are now largely below 100 $\mu g/m^3$ [2], having declined from an earlier range of 100-200 $\mu g/m^3$ [84]. There has also been a decline in maximum daily mean values to the current 250-500 $\mu g/m^3$ range, while peaks over shorter averaging periods (e.g., 1 hour) extend to 1,000-2,000 $\mu g/m^3$ or higher [2]. The annual mean SO_2 concentrations in most rural areas of Europe are between 5-25 $\mu g/m^3$, although, due to the use of high chimneys to disperse emissions, there are also large rural areas in Europe where average concentrations of SO_2 exceed 25 $\mu g/m^3$ [2]. In the U.S., nationwide SO_2 emissions in 1985 were 23 million tons, and 56% of these emissions were vented through smoke stacks taller than 145 meters, which enabled these pollutants to travel long distances [82].

Sulphuric Acid (Acid Aerosol)

Sulphuric acid is the most irritant of the S(VI) aerosols present in the atmosphere. Levels of sulphuric acid reported range from 20 ng/m^3 to 240 $\mu g/m^3$ [86]. Ranges of 20-30 μg sulphuric acid/m^3 (6-12 hours average) in various part of North America, and 28 μg sulphuric acid/m^3 in Europe (West Berlin) have been reported [87]. The highest reported level in the UK was 680 μg sulphuric acid/m^3 (1-hour average) in London in 1962. However, higher levels are believed to have been present in London in earlier years [20].

Rates of SO_2 oxidation depend on various factors, including ambient temperature, humidity, concentrations of oxidants and catalytic components of particles in the atmosphere and cloud droplets [2].

Sulphur (VI), as well as trace metals capable of promoting the oxidation of SO_2 to H_2SO_4, are concentrated in the sub-μm fraction of atmospheric aerosols and of ash from coal combustion. With certain coals, as much as 9% of the sulphur present in the coal was detected in the ultrafine (0.1 μm) ash fraction as either free H_2SO_4 or as a surface layer on the particles. Sulphur and the relevant trace metals are concentrated on the surface of particles emitted from power plants and electrical steel furnaces. The ultrafine metal oxide and SO_2 have been postulated to react during coal combustion or smelting operations to form primary emissions coated with an acidic SO_x layer [86].

Carbon Monoxide

Carbon monoxide is one of the most common and widely distributed air pollutants; its total emissions into the atmosphere are believed to equal or exceed those of all other air pollutants combined [2]. Estimates of CO emission vary from 350 to 600 million tons/year, with the principal sources of emissions resulting from incomplete combustion processes (e.g., in vehicles, industrial processes, heating facilities and incinerators). Additionally, CO is produced by natural sources as well as chemical reactions in the troposphere and biosphere processes [2-5]. The principal biosphere CO production processes are based on the oxidation from plant material, photooxidation of organic matter in ocean water, and chemical oxidation of organic carbon in soil. In addition, there is evidence that CO is produced by biological reduction of CO_2 due to the activity of anaerobic bacteria (e.g., sulphate-reducing bacteria), methanogenic bacteria and acetogenic bacteria [88].

Natural background levels of CO range between 0.01 and 0.23 mg/m^3 (0.01-0.20 ppm). Concentrations in urban areas are according to time and distance from the sources. Although 8-hour mean concentrations are generally less than 20 mg/m^3 (17 ppm), maximum 8-hour mean concentrations of up to 60 mg/m^3 (53 ppm) have been reported [2].

Carbonyl Compounds

Carbonyl compounds, including aldehydes and ketones, are found in urban and industrial atmospheres as primary pollutants. They also occur in the atmosphere as secondary pollutants, that is, they arise as the products of the first stage of photo-oxidation of organic compounds. Carbonyl compounds (except formaldehyde) are the direct precursors of peroxyacyl nitrates in the atmosphere. Carbonyl compounds (principally formaldehyde) are, via their photolysis, promoters of free radicals whose importance becomes preponderant in moderately or highly polluted atmospheres [89], and are formed in all emission sources.

Formaldehyde and acetaldehyde are the most abundant carbonyl compounds in the atmosphere, although significant fractions of total carbonyls (about 10%) may be present as acetone, acrolein, propanal, and benzaldehyde. Aldehydes are formed through photooxidation reactions of methane and isoprene and other biogenic and anthropogenic hydrocarbons. In the industrialised areas of the world, aldehydes (as well as ketones) are also directly emitted during manufacturing processes and via transportation (vehicular) sources. In general, the lifetimes of aldehydes are in the order of hours, with the principal gas-phase loss routes by photolysis and reaction with OH radicals (estimated to cause a daily loss rate of about 80% of atmospheric acetaldehyde emissions).

Formaldehyde and Acetaldehyde

Formaldehyde and acetaldehyde atmosphere levels are especially important since these derivatives substantially influence photochemical smog processes in complex ways, e.g. by accelerating the formation of secondary products and increasing ozone maxima. Gas-phase photolysis of formaldehyde in the atmosphere can lead, via reaction with OH or via photolysis, to the net formation of 1 or 2 hydroperoxyl (HO_2) radicals. These radicals can oxidise nitric oxide (NO) molecules to NO_2 and OH or recombine to yield hydrogen peroxide. Photolysis of acetaldehyde in the atmosphere leads to the formation of HO_2 radicals, CO and methyl peroxyl radicals and, by reaction with OH, to the peroxyacetyl radical and peroxyacetyl nitrate (PAN). In polluted urban air, day-time decomposition of acetaldehyde via reaction with OH is expected to be a major route of PAN formation, especially away from the immediate vicinity of the NO emission source [90].

Although formaldehyde occurs in air from natural environment (as an intermediary in the methane cycle with low background concentrations), the major sources are anthropogenic, including direct emissions (the production and use of formaldehyde) and secondary reactions of oxidised hydrocarbons from stationary and mobile sources (automobile exhaust, combustion processes in power plants, petroleum refineries, incinerators) [2,72]. Automobile exhaust itself contains formaldehyde at concentrations of 29-48 ppm (35.7-52.9 mg/m^3), and this source has been reported to account for much of the formaldehyde present in the atmosphere [72]. The natural background concentration of formaldehyde is a few μg/m^3. In urban air, the annual average is approximately 0.005-0.01 mg/m^3, with higher levels in the vicinity of industrial processes. Concentrations of formaldehyde are about one order of magnitude greater during short-term peaks occurring at peak traffic periods in built-up urban areas or under photochemical smog conditions [2,72]. Ambient levels of formaldehyde in the range of 5-60 ppb have typically been reported in polluted atmospheres in the U.S.; acetaldehyde levels are in the order of 60% of formaldehyde levels [90]. In Switzerland, concentrations of 9.3-10 ppb (11.4-12.3 $\mu g/m^3$) formaldehyde in street air and levels of 0.1-6.5 ppb (0.12-8 $\mu g/m^3$) in maritime air in the northern part of the Federal Republic of Germany have been reported [72]. The use of ethanol-based fuels as a constituent in gasohol (20% v/v in normal usage) and in pure form as a fuel in a smaller portion (10-15%) of vehicles with engines designed to burn hydrated ethanol and with no catalytic controls (as utilised in Brazil), has led to increased primary emissions and high ambient levels of formaldehyde, acetaldehyde and other higher aldehydes in polluted urban air. Analogous recent proposed use of methanol-based fuel (15% v/v in normal usage) or in pure form as a fuel in specially designed vehicles in the U.S. has been shown to lead to elevated primary emissions and higher ambient levels of formaldehyde.

The major anthropogenic sources of formaldehyde affecting humans are to be found in indoor environments with primary sources including insulating materials, chipboard, plywood fabrics as well as from heating, cooling and cigarette smoke [2,8,12,72].

Acetaldehyde occurs in air as a result of natural and anthropogenic sources, with the latter being by far the greatest source. The annual U.S. atmospheric emissions of acetaldehyde in 1978 were initially reported to range from 2.2-12.2 million kg/yr. A more detailed estimation of 52 million kg in 1978 from all sources (80% of which was due to wood burning in residences) was later reported [91]. The major manufacturing sources included: coffee roasting, acetic acid, vinyl acetate, ethanol, acrylonitrile and crotonaldehyde. Air monitoring data between 1975 and 1978 showed mean ambient concentrations of 5-124 $\mu g/m^3$ acetaldehyde at 7 U.S. locations. It has also been detected in ambient air in Southern California under conditions of moderate to severe photochemical pollution at levels of 5.4-62 $\mu g/m^3$ [91], and in air near and in a refuse-reclamation area in Japan at levels of 5.4-13.7 $\mu g/m^3$ [91].

Organochlorine Pesticides and Polychlorinated Biphenyls

A broad spectrum of halogenated hydrocarbons representing predominately organochloro pesticides and the polychlori-nated biphenyls (PCBs) are emitted into the atmosphere via direct industrial, commercial, agricultural and residential emissions, evaporation from contaminated waters, soils or vegetative surfaces, or re-enter the atmosphere by processes such as volatisation or resuspension [92].

In urban and rural localities, hexachlorobenzene (HCB) concentrations are reported to be within the range of 0.2-0.3 ng/m^3, while lindane concentrations are in the range of 0.02-7 ng/m^3. Background concentrations in remote marine atmospheres are reported to be within a range of 0.03-0.23 ng/m^3 for HCB and 0.01-5 ng/m^3 for lindane [93].

The atmospheric transport and deposition of several classes of chlorinated organic compounds such as the polychlorinated biphenyls (PCBs) and pesticides, is regarded as an important pathway for the input of these contaminants to the Great Lakes, oceans and even to the most remote regions of the globe [93-95]. Samples of peat, bogs and Arctic snow attest to the atmospheric transport and subsequent wet and dry deposition of halogenated organic compounds (primarily organochlorine pesticides) such as hexachlorocyclohexanes (HCH), lindane, alpha and gamma chlordane, heptachlor, DDT, toxaphene, hexachlorobenzene (HCB) and polychlorinated biphenyls (PCBs) [94,95]. In a study of peat cores in the mid-latitudes of North America, the input (source functions) derived from peat profiles was consistent with production and use information in the the U.S. for PCBs, hexachlorobenzene, hexachloroclohexanes, DDT and toxaphene [95].

The distribution of atmospheric PCBs between vapour phase, aerosols and rain was recently elaborated by Duinker and Bouchertall [96], who separated PCB congeners in filtered air, in particulates and in rain collected simultaneously in an urban area in the Federal Republic of Germany. The PCB mixture was dominated by congeners with a low degree of chlorination in the filtered air, by congeners with a high degree of chlorination in the aerosols and in rain. The vapour phase represented up to 99% of total atmospheric concentrations for the most volatile congeners. Particle scavenging was the dominant source of PCBs in rain, despite the small contribution (only 1 or 2%) of particulate PCBs to the total atmospheric concentration. Little information is available on the chemical reactivity of the organochlorine pesticides and PCBs under tropospheric conditions. The major chemical reaction for many of these compounds in the troposphere appears to be with hydroxyl radicals.

Polychlorinated Dibenzo-p-Dioxins and Polychlorinated Dibenzofurans

Polychlorinated dibenzo-p-dioxins (PCDDS) and polychlorinated dibenzofurans (PCDFs) are of increasing toxicological and environmental concern, principally with regard to the ubiquity in the environment and suspected carcinogenicity of specific isomers of these 2 important classes of chlorinated derivatives. There are 75 isomers of the PCDDs and 135 PCDF isomers, of which 2,3,7,8-tetra-chlorodibenzo-p-dioxin (TCDD) is by far the most toxic of all the isomers of PCDDs and PCDFs. Toxicities can vary by a factor of 1,000 to 10,000 for isomers as closely related as 2,3,7,8-and 1,2,3,4-TCDD and 1,2,4,7,8-pentachlorodibenzodioxin. PCDDs and PCDFs are released into the environment, e.g., atmosphere, via the improper disposal of contaminated production wastes and incineration or other high-temperature processes. Certain congeners are extremely stable compounds which, once released, are persistent in the environment [97,98].

The distribution of PCDDs and PCDfs in combustion effluents and soots has been examined [98]. While there are many combustion sources of PCDDs and PCDFs, one notable source is thermal events ("fires") in electrical equipment containing dielectric fluid (mixtures of PCBs and trichlorobenzene). These thermal events can be explosions, fires, electrical arcs and thermal evaporation. Another source of airborne chlorinated dioxins and dibenzofurans of increasing concern arises from the incineration of municipal and hazardous wastes, and in the U.S. also from Superfund site cleanup operations [97]. Recent studies have shown the presence of numerous PCDD/PCDF congeners in Swedish, Danish and Canadian incinerator wastes with virtually all the congeners present [99]. The 2,3,7,8-TCDD congener was always present as a minor constituent, whereas in all samples 1,2,3,7,8-penta-CDD

was a peak of "medium" size. The toxic hexa-CDDs and CDFs were always medium or major components. A striking similarity in the pattern of PCDDs and PCDFs was found between samples from different incinerators. Hutzinger et al. [100] suggested that about 3-4% of the total PCDD stack emissions near municipal incinerators may be tetrachloro isomers, of which about 5% could be 2,3,7,8-TCDD.

Measurable amounts of a large number of PCDDs and PCDFs have been found in urban air. The highest levels measured were about 5-10 picograms/m^3 for the sum of all PCDDs an PCDFs. In suburban areas the levels were a factor of 5-10 lower [101].

Hydrochloric Acid

The major anthropogenic hydrochloric acid emissions to the atmosphere arise from burning material containing chloride, principally fuels. In the United Kingdom, coal is the largest single source of HCl emissions. The mean chloride content of British coal is 0.23% and it has been estimated that 99% of this is most probably emitted as HCl in stack gases during combustion. The total annual HCl emission in the U.K. is estimated to be 240 k tons, based on coal delivery in the U.K. of 1.12 x 10^5 kt in 1983. The estimated total emission of HCl from 12 other West European countries is about 380 k tons/year [102].

Other sources of HCl to the atmosphere include the incineration of domestic and industrial waste, where HCl arises from chlorides in material such as vegetable matter, paper, polyvinyl chloride (PVC) plastic, dry cell batteries and salt. It is estimated that waste incineration accounts for about 16 k tons/year HCl to the atmosphere, of which approximately 8 k tons arise from HCl emissions from PVC waste in municipal incinerators. In the U.K., coal burning and waste incineration account for about 99% of HCl emissions [102].

Industrial sources of HCl are relatively small compared with emissions from coal burning and waste incineration and include glass manufacture and production of steel (steel pickling acid and regeneration). In the Federal Republic of Germany, power stations and industrial furnaces produced 81.4% of HCl emissions, waste incineration produced

17.5% and other sources only 1.1% [103]. Another potential anthropogenic source of atmosphere HCl arises from the production and use of chlorinated hydrocarbons which are released into the atmosphere as solvents, refrigerants etc., and which react very slowly in the atmosphere to yield HCl. In the U.K., the chlorinated hydrocarbons represent a potential HCl source of about 400 k tons/year. However, it should be noted that the atmospheric reactions of chlorinated hydrocarbon with OH radicals to produce HCl is so slow that the acidity produced as HCl is well dispersed over the Northern hemisphere and is considered not distinguishable from the background acidity of the atmosphere. Natural sources may also be an important source of atmospheric hydrochloric acid. For example, HCl is emitted from volcanoes and the total world emissions from this source, although very uncertain, has been estimated to range from 750 k tons/yr to 7,600 tons/year. An additional source of HCl in the atmosphere is methyl chloride which is produced in the sea by marine plants or microorganisms and also on land via the combustion of vegetation. Methyl chloride in the atmosphere reacts with OH radicals and the chloride content is eventually converted to HCl. Globally it has been estimated that natural sources produce 5,600 k tons of methylchloride per year, which is equivalent to about 400 k tons of HCl.

Molina et al. [104] recently suggested that the observed depletion of ozone over Antarctica could in some measure be accounted for by the reaction between atmospheric hydrogen chloride and chlorine nitrate ($ClO NO_2$), which is greatly enhanced in the presence of ice particles. This reaction has 2 important effects: it promotes the formation of HNO_3 with the corresponding depression of NO_2, and it generates Cl_2, which photolyses rapidly to produce catalytically active free radicals that may rapidly destroy ozone in the absence of high NO_2 levels.

Ammonia and Ammonium

Ammonia and ammonium are important atmospheric components. The main sources of NH_3 are predominantly emissions from the livestock wastes and to a lesser degree from fertiliser application. Fertiliser factories also yield localised emissions and other small contributions arise from traffic and coal combustion.

The spatial distribution of annual emissions in England and Wales summed over different sources amount to approximately 300 k tons/year, with that of Scotland amounting to about 70 k tons/year. Studies of longer-term trends imply a 50% increase in NH_3 emissions over Europe between 1950 and 1980 [105]. Ammonia is suggested to be the only significant gaseous atmospheric trace species capable of neutralising airborne acidity. In this process, it converts strong acids to relatively neutral ammonium salt aerosols. Atmospheric concentrations of ammonia and ammonium are typically in the order of a few micrograms/m^3 and may be subject to seasonal and rapid temporal variations [106]. Ammonia is important for aerosol nitrate formation. Large emissions of NH_3 can lead to high concentrations of $NH_4 NO_3$ (e.g., as over the East Los Angeles Basin). Thus, ammonia can have an important role in altering oxidation and pollutant deposition systematically on a regional basis and is involved in the acid rain problem [105].

Asbestos

Asbestos is the generic name for a group of naturally occurring mineral silicate fibres of serpentine and amphibole series. The principal varieties of asbestos are chrysotile, crocidolite, amosite, anthophyllite, tremolite and actinolite. Although chrysotile is a reasonably well defined mineral, the 5 amphibole asbestiform fibres possess variable chemical compositions. The asbestos fibres are bundles of thinner fibres made up of fibrils which, in the case of chrysotile, have a diameter of 20-25 nm [2]. Emissions of asbestos result from natural weathering as well as mining and milling, manufacture of products, construction activities, transport and use of asbestos-containing products, removal and disposal. Additional sources of asbestos emissions occur during processing, rain acidity which can corrode asbestos-cement sheets and from the wear of vehicle brake linings [2,107,108].

Asbestos fibres of respirable size form part of a range of fibrous aerosols in the lower atmosphere. (Other fibres include man-made mineral fibres, fibrous silica and aluminum oxide, fibrous gypsum etc. [2].) Asbestos fibres may travel considerable distances in the atmosphere because of their aerodynamic properties and since no chemical decomposition of the fibres occur, the only cleaning mechanism is via washout or by rain or snow [2].

The general levels of asbestos found in urban areas vary from 100 to 1,000 fibres (F)/m^3 [2,108,109] and below 100 F/m^3 in rural areas remote from asbestos emission sources [2,110]. Although levels of asbestos fibres in occupational settings are often much higher by orders of magnitude than those found in environmental settings (e.g., 10^5 F/m^3 to more than 10^8 F/m^3, they are now being reduced to below 2 x 10^6 F/m^3 in most countries and to (0.2 - 0.5) x 10^6 F/m^3 in some countries [2,111]. It should also be noted that indoor asbestos fibre concentrations can be considerably higher than outdoor concentrations principally resulting from the friability of asbestos insulation material (e.g., asbestos/plastors, spray asbestos, asbestos cement etc.). While in buildings without specific asbestos sources, concentrations are generally below 100F/m^3, in buildings with friable asbestos, exposures can reach 10,000 F/m^3 [2].

Silica

The term silica is used to refer to naturally occurring materials (in both crystalline and amorphous forms) composed principally of silicon dioxide (SiO_2) with the greater majority of natural crystalline SiO_2 existing as quartz [112]. Three crystalline, polymorphic forms are most relevant to human health: quartz, tridymite and cristobalite. Although there is an extensive literature on specific workplace exposure levels in many countries dealing with mining and quarrying, ceramics, glass and related industries, very much less data is available on atmospheric levels of silica either on a local, national or global basis [112].

Local conditions, especially in deserts and areas near recent volcanic eruptions and mine dumps, can give rise to airborne silica-containing dust. Data on "free silica" in air is generally derived indirectly. Quantities of airborne dust originating from world deserts have been estimated to be 4.5 x 10^8 tons, which are shifted annually to new depositional sites. The mineral varieties range considerably and are only in part silica [112].

Suspended Particulate Matter

The generic classification "atmospheric particulates' includes an enormous variety of inorganic and organic substances that can be generated from both natural and anthropogenic sources. Hence, individual particles can be composed of different chemicals, and can be homogenous or heterogenous in their structure as well as vary in their size and shape. Particle size has been principally employed as the single most important parameter in specifying the composition of airborne particulate matter and, because of the complexity of particulate matter, multiple terms (e.g., suspended particulate matter, total suspended particulates, black smoke, as well as terms referring to the site of deposition in the respirable tract) are often used [2]. Mass and composition of particulate matter can be divided in 2 main groups: coarse particles larger than 2.5 µm air aerodynamic diameter and fine particles smaller than 2.5 µm in aerodynamic diameter. The natural sources of particulate matter include volcanoes and dust storms, while the more widespread and important sources are anthropogenic (e.g., vehicular traffic, domestic coal burning, power plants, industrial processes and incinerators) [2,4,5,8,10,11].

Since the early 1980s, there has been an increased utilisation of diesel engines in both light and heavy duty motor vehicles and of coal for power generation and heating in many countries; this has been manifest in the increasingly heavy burden of atmospheric fine particulates as well as gaseous NO_x and SO_x in major urban areas throughout the world [10,111,54]. Organic compounds absorbed in the particulate phase of petrol and diesel exhausts have been studied extensively. Diesel particulate organic matter (POM) is emitted in the submicron, respiratory size range (<0.5µm) and comparable to most combustion-generated particulates, contains a number of promutagenic and carcinogenic PAHs as well as other unidentified mutagens that exhibit strong direct activity in the Ames Salmonella/mammalian microsome assay [10,11,54,113,114]. The characterisation of organic particulate mixtures is acknowledged to be extremely difficult. Urban air particles contain extractable organic matter that has been shown on many occasions to possess mutagenic and carcinogenic activity. The concentrations of PAHs in the particulate phase of ambient air have been studied extensively [10,11,18]. The ratio of PAHs in the vapour and particulate phases of the samples monitored has been shown to vary considerably with traffic, season and meteorological conditions [18]. A large number of PAHs have been isolated from particulates emitted in diesel exhausts. These include: phenanthrene, fluoranthene, pyrene, benzo(ghi)fluoranthene, cyclopenteno(cd)pyrene, benz(a)-anthracene, chrysene, benzo(a)pyrene, benzo(e)pyrene, indeno(1,2,3-ed) pyrene, benzo(ghi) pyrene and coronene [115,116].

The nitro-PAHs that have been found in diesel particulates include: nitrofluorenes, nitroanthracenes, nitrophenanthrenes, nitrofluoranthenes, nitropyrene, and methylnitro (pyrene and fluoranthenes) and are believed to account for a major portion of the direct acting mutagenicity of diesel particulates [54,116]. Many mutagenic chemical fractions of diesel particulate extracts have been found to contain oxygenated PAH derivatives, including compounds with hydroxy, ketone, quinone, carboxaldehyde, acid anhydride, dihydroxy and acid substituents on the parent PAH [116].

Chemical and physical transformations may occur in the presence of sunlight and oxygen, and cover a spectrum of copollutants (e.g., HONO, $HONO_2$, PAN, and the nitrate radical, NO_3) during transport of wood smoke and diesel particulate organic matter and NO_x in the atmosphere over periods of hours or days or even weeks.

Another principal source of atmospheric particulates arises from metallic elements in fossil fuel combustion products. Of some 80 elements that are considered as metals, about 50 have been reported to be present in coal, 35 in crude oil, 30 in fuel oil and about 20 in petrol. As a result of combustion, these elements are mobilised and may be emitted into the atmosphere primarily as constituents of particulate matter containing a mixture of inorganic and organic substances [117]. The composition and structure of these particulate emissions depend on the fuel and the combustion processes employed. Combustion of fossil fuels in electric power plants, commercial boilers and furnaces for space heating, and in motor vehicles, is the principle anthropogenic source of metallic elements in the atmosphere. Metallic elements mobilised by coal combustion are partitioned between the slag or bottom ash and fly ash with some metals temporarily remaining in the gaseous state. During combustion, the chalcophile elements (e.g., those which readily form sulphides), are volatilised and later condensed onto the surface of fly ash particles. Since the surface area per unit mass increases with decreasing particle size, the concentration of metallic elements increases in the submicron (respirable) range of particle size [117]. The levels of suspended particulate matter are increasing in the urban atmosphere of the developing countries [85].

REFERENCES

1   Graedel TE, Hawkins DT, Claxton LD: Atmospheric compounds: merging the chemical and bioassay data. In: Graedel TE, Hawkins DT and Claxton LD (eds) Atmospheric Chemical Compounds. Academic Press, Orlando 1986 pp1-42

2   Quality Guidelines for Europe. WHO Regional Publications. European Series No. 23. World Health Organization - Regional Office for Europe, Copenhagen 1987 p 410

3   Seinfeld TH: Urban air pollution: state of the science. Science 1989 (243):745-752

4   Ember LR, Layman PL, Lepkowski W, Zurer PS: Tending to global commons. Chem Eng News 1986 (Nov. 24):14-64

5   McElroy MB, Salawitch RJ: Changing composition of the global stratosphere. Science 1989 (243):763-770

6   Nriagu JO, Pacyna JM: Quantitative assessment of worldwide contamination of air, water and soil by trace metals. Nature 1988 (333):134-139

7   Lloy PJ, Daisey JM: Airborne toxic elements and organic substances. Environ Sci Technol 1985 (20):8-1

8   Shah JJ, Sing HB: Distribution of volatile organic chemicals in outdoor and indoor air. Environ Sci Technol 1988 (22):1383-1388

9   Graham JD, Green LC, Roberts MJ: In Search of Safety-Chemicals and Cancer Risk. Harvard Univ Press, Cambridge MA 1988.

10   Lewtas J: Combustion emissions: characterization and comparison of their mutagenic and carcinogenic activity: In: Stich H (ed) Carcinogens and Mutagens in the Environment. Vol 5. CRC Press, Boca Ration, FL, 1985 pp 60-74

11   Lewtas SJ, Gallagher J: Identification and comparative assessment of mutagenic and tumorigenic chemicals and emission sources. In: Proceedings of Experimental and Epidemiologic Applications to Risk Assessment of Complex Mixtures, Espoo, Finland, June 14-17

12   Lewtas J: Toxicology of complex mixtures of indoor air pollutants. Ann Rev Pharmacol Toxicol 1989 (29):415-439

13   Schroeder WH, Lane DA: The fate of toxic airborne pollutants. Environ Sci Technol 1988 (22):240-246

14   Schwartz SE: Acid deposition: unraveling a regional phenomenon. Science 1989 (243):753-763

15   Anon: reducing acid rain - continuation of the Pimental report. Environ Sci Technol 1985 (29):439-440

16   Anon: Tougher laws on toxic emissions urged. Chem Eng News 1989 (April 3):23-24

17   U.S. House of Representatives: The National Toxic Release Inventory-Preliminary Air Toxic Data. Washington, DC. Subcommittee on Health and the Environment, Committee on Energy and Commerce. 1989 (March 22): p 78

18   Tuominen S, Salomaa S, Pyysalo H, Skytta E: Polynuclear aromatic compounds and genotoxicity in particulate and vapor phases of ambient air: effect to traffic, season and meterological conditions. Environ Sci Technol 1988 (22):1228-1234

19   Merian E: Introduction on enviornmental chemistry and global cycles of chromium, nickel, cobalt, beryllium, arsenic, cadmium and selenium and their derivatives. Toxicol Environ Chem 1984 (8):9-38

20   Lee RE, Von Lehmden, DJ: Trace metal pollution and the environment J Air Pollut Control Assoc 1973 (73):853-862

21   Lee RE, Duffield FV: Some sources of environmentally important metals in the atmosphere. Adv Chem Ser 1977(170):42-55

22   Natusch DFS, Wallace JR, Evans CA: Toxic trace elements: preferential concentration in respirable particles. Science 1974 (183):202-209

23   U.S. Environmental Protection Agency: National Emissions Report, EPA-450/2-76-007. Research Triangle Park, N.C.1973 (May)

24   Chadwick MJ, Highton NN, Lindman M: Environmental impacts of coal mining and utilization. Pergamon Press, Oxford 1978 pp197-198

25   Chilvers DC, Peterson PJ: Global cycling of arsenic. In: Hutchinson TC and Meema RM (eds) Lead, Mercury, Cadmium and Arsenic in the Environment. John Wiley & Sons, Chichester, UK 1987 pp 279-302

26   Hutton M, Wadge A, Mulligan PH: Environmental levels of cadmium and lead in the vicinity of a major refuse incinerator. Atmos Environ 1988 (22):411-416

27   Greenberg RR, Zoller WH, Gordon GE: Composition and size distribution of particles released in refuse incineration. Environ Sci Technol 1978 (12):560-569

28   Fishbein L: Potential metal toxicity from hazardous waste incineration. Toxicol Environ Chem 1989 (18):287-309

29   Wadge AM Hutton M: The cadmium and lead content of suspended particulate matter emitted from a U.K. refuse incinerator. Sci Total Environ 1987 (67):91-88

30   Lantzy RJ, Mackenzie FT: Atmospheric trace metals: global cycles and assessment of man's impact. Geochim Cosmochim Acta 1979 (43):511-525

31   Nriagru JO: Global inventory of natural and anthropogenic emissions of trace metals to the atmosphere. Nature 1979 (279):409-411

32   Pacyna JM: In Hutchinson TC and Meema KM (eds) Lead, Mercury, Cadmium and Arsenic in the Environment. John Wiley & Sons, Chichester, UK 1987 pp 69-87

33   Peters JM, Thomas D, Falk H, Oberdoster G, Smith TJ: Contribution of Metals to Respiratory Cancer. Environ Hlth Persp 1986 (70):71-83

34   Zacharewski TR, Cherniak EA, Schroeder WH: FTIR Investigation of the heterogeneous reaction of HgO with SO_2 at ambient temperature. Atmos Environ 1987 (21):2327-2332

35   Lahmann E et al: Heavy Metals: Identification of Air Quality and Environmental Problems in the European Community. Vol. 1 and 2. (Report No. Eur 10678 EN/I and Eur 10678 En/II). Luxembourg, Commission of the European Communities 1986

36 Radojevic M, Harrison RM: Concentration, speciation and decomposition of organo lead compounds in rain water. Atmos Environ 1987 (21):2403-2411

37 Hewitt CN, Harrison RM: Atmospheric concentrations and chemistry of alkyl lead compounds and environmental alkylation of ead. Environ Sci Technol 1987 (21):360-266

38 UNEP/WHO: Lead: Environmental Health Criteria 3. Geneva, United Nations Environment Programme/World Health Organization: 21-27, 30-42, 44-68, 80-86

39 National Academy of Sciences: Biological Effects of Atmospheric Pollutants. Lead: Airborne Lead In Perspective. Washington, DC, National Research Council: 5-84, 131-144, 178-191, 226-248

40 IARC: IARC Monographs on the Evaluation of the Carcinogenic Risk of Chemicals to Humans. Vol. 23. Some Metals and Metallic Compounds. International Agency for Research on Cancer, Lyon 1980 pp 242,243,344-345.

41 Nriagu JO: Lead in the atmosphere. In: Nriagu JO (ed) The Biogeochemistry of Lead in the Environment. Part A. Elsevier-North Holland, Amsterdam 1978 pp 137-184

42 Fishbein L: Environmental metallic carcinogens: an overview of exposure levels. J Toxicol Env Hlth 1976 (2):77-109

43 EPA: Health Assessment Document For Chromium. Final Report No. EPA-600/8-83-014 F. Research Triangle Park, NC U.S. Environmental Protection Agency

44 Bowen HJM: Environmental Chemistry of the Elements. Academic Press, London 1979

45 EPA: Health Assessment for Nickel. Report No. EPA-7--/8-83-012F. Research Triangle Park, N.C. U.S. Environmental Protection Agency

46 Schmidt JA, Andren AW: The atmospheric chemistry of nickel. In: Nriagu JO: (ed) Nickel in the Environment. John Wiley & Sons, New York 1980 pp 93-135.

47 National Research Council of Canada: Effects of Nickel in the Canadian Environment. Report No. 18568, Ottawa 1981

48 Behymer TD, Hites RA: Photolysis of polycyclic aromatic hydrocarbons absorbed on fly ash. Environ Sci Technol 1988 (22):1311-1319

49 National Academy of Sciences: Polycyclic Aromatic Hydrocarbons: Evaluation of Sources and Effects. Washington, DC, National Research Council 1983

50 IARC: IARC Monographs on the Carcinogenic Risk of Chemicals to Humans. Vol 32. Polynuclear Aromatic Compounds. Part 1. Chemical, Environmental and Experimental Data. International Agency for Research on Cancer, Lyon 1983

51 Ahland E et al: Air Pollution and Cancer. Investigation of hazardous constituents from various emission sources for their carcinogenic impact. Münchener Med Wochenschr 1985 (127):218-221

52 Pott F: Pyrolytic profiles of polycyclic aromatic hydrocarbons and lung cancer risk - data evaluation. Staubreinhalt Luft 1985 (45):369-379

53 Pitts JN Jr: Nitration of gaseous polyaromatic hydrocarbons in simulated and ambient urban atmospheres: a source of mutagenic nitroarenes. Atmos Environ 1987 (21):2531-2547

54 Pitts JN Jr: Formation and fate of gaseous and particulate mutagens and carcinogens in real and simulated atmospheres. Environ Hlth Persp 1983 (47):115-140

55 Pitts JN Jr, Van Cawenberghe KA, Grosjean, D, Schmid JP: Atmospheric reaction of PAH: facile formation of mutagenic nitro derivatives. Science 1978 (202):515-521

56 Arey J, Atkinson R, Zielinska B, McElroy PA: Diurnal concentrations of volatile polycyclic aromatic hydrocarbons and nitroarenes during a photochemical air pollution episode in Glenodra, California. Environ Sci Technol 1989 (23):321-327

57 Singh HB, Hanst PL: Peroxyacetyl Nitrate (PAN) in the unpolluted atmosphere: an important reservoir for nitrogen oxides. Geophys Res Lett 1981 (8):941-946

58 Rogers JD, Rhead LA: Peroxyglutaryl Nitrate Formation and Infrared Spectrum. Atmos Environ 1987 (21):2519-2522

59 Schuetle D, Cronn D, Crittenden AC, Carlson RJ: Molecular composition of secondary aerosol and its possible origin. Environ Sci Technol 1975 (9):838-845

60 Walcek CJ: A Theoretical estimate of O_3 and H_2O_2 dry deposition over the Northeast United States. Atmos Environ 1987 (21):2649-2659

61 Hartkamph, Bachhawsen P: A method for the determination of hydrogen peroxide in air. Atmos Environ 1987 (21):2207-2213

62 Hileman B: Global Warming. Chem Eng News 1989 (March 13):25-44

63 Killus JP, Whitten GZ: Isoprene: A photochemical kinetic mechanism. Environ Sci Technol 1984 (18):142-148

64 Scheere KL: Modeling ozone concentrations. Environ Sci Technol 1988 (22):488-495

65 EPA: Air quality criteria for ozone and other photochemical oxidants. 4 Volumes. Report No. EPA-600/8-84-02F. Washington, D.C. U.S. Environmental Protection Agency 1986

66 Zurer P: U.S. seeks tighter rules on ozone protection. Chem Eng News 1989 (May 1):8-9

67 Graedel TE, Crutzen PJ: The changing atmosphere. Sci Amer 1989 (261):508-608

68 Charles D: EPA's plan for cooling the global greenhouse. Science 1989 (243):1542-1543

69 Graedel TE: Hydrocarbons. In: Graedel TE, Hawkins DT and Claxton LD (eds) Atmospheric Chemical Compounds. Academic Press, Orlando 1986 pp 11-298

70 IARC: IARC Monographs on the Evaluation of the Carcinogenic Risk of Chemicals to Humans. Vol 19. Some Monomers, Plastics and Synthetic Elastomers, and Acrolein. International Agency for Research on Cancer, Lyon 1979 pp 157-186; 213-230

71 IARC: IARC Monographs on the Evaluation of the Carinogenic Risk of Chemicals to Humans. Vol 19. Some Monomers, Plastics and Synthetic

Elastomers, and Acrolein. International Agency for Research on Cancer, Lyon 1985 pp 155-179

72 IARC: IARC Monographs on the Evaluation of the Carcinogenic Risk of Chemicals to Humans. Vol 39. Some Industrial Chemicals and Dyestuffs. International Agency for Research on Cancer, Lyon 1982 pp 93-148

73 Merian E, Znader M: Volatile Aromatics. In: Hutzinger O (ed) Handbook of Environmental Chemistry. Vol 3, Part B, Anthropogenic Compounds. Springer-Verlag, Berlin 1982 pp 117-161

74 EPA: Ambient Air, Water Quality Criteria for Benzene. Epa-440/5-80-018. Washington, D.C. U.S. Environmental Protection Agency. 1980:C1-C8, C16-C35, C68-C100

75 Korte F, Klein W: Degradation of benzene in the environment. Ecotox. Environ Saf 1982 (6):311-327

76 IARC: IARC Monographs on the Evaluation of the Carcinogenic Risk of Chemicals to Humans. Vol 41. Some Halogenated Hydrocarbons and Pesticide Exposures. International Agency for Research on Cancer, Lyon 1986 pp 161-186

77 Edwards PR, Campbell, I, Milne GS: The impact of chloromethanes on the environment. Part 2. Methylchloride and methylene chloride. Chem Ind 1982 (17):619-622

78 Singh HB, Salas LJ, Smith AJ, Shigeishi H: Measurements of some potentially hazardous organic chemicals in urban environments. Atmos Environ 1981 (15):601-612

79 Singh HB, Salas LJ, Stiles RE: Distribution of selected gaseous organic mutagens and suspect carcinogens in ambient air. Environ Sci Technol 1982 (16):872-880

80 Janssen LH, Van Wakeren JH, Van Duuren H, Elshout AJ: A classification of NO oxidation rates in power plant plumes based on atmospheric conditions. Atmos Environ 1988 (22):43-53

81 EPA: Air Quality Criteria for Oxides of Nitrogen. Report No. EPA-600/8-82-026F. Research Triangle Park, NC, U.S. Environmental Protection Agency 1982

82 Anon: California, Indiana, Ohio and Texas allegedly are the highest emitters of acid rain precursors. Environ Sci Technol 1989 (23):375

83 EPA: Air Quality Criteria for Particulate Matter and Sulfur Oxides. Vols. I-II (EPA-600/8-82-029 a,b,c). Research Triangle Park NC, US Environmental Protection Agency 1982

84 WHO: Sulfur oxides and Suspended Particulate Matter. Environmental Health Criteria No. 8. World Health Organization, Geneva 1979

85 UNEP: Environmental Data Report 1989-1990. Basic Blackwell, Oxford 1989

86 Amdur MO, Sarofim AF, Neville M, Quann PJ, McCarthy JF: Coal combustion, aerosols and SO_2: an interdisciplinary Aanalysis. Environ Sci Technol 1986 (20):138-145

87 Lloy PJ, Lippmann M: Measurements of exposure to acidic sulfur aerosols. In: Lee SD et al (eds) Aerosols. Lewis, Chelsea MI 1986

88 Conrad R, Schutz H, Seller W: Emission of carbon monoxide from submerged rice fields into the atmosphere. Atmos Environ 1988 (2):821-823

89 Kalabokas P, Carlier P, Fresnet P, Mouvier G, Toupance G: Field studies of aldehyde chemistry in the Paris area. Atmos Environ 1988 (22):147-155

90 Tanner RL, Miguel AH, de Andrade JB, Gaffney JS, Streit GE: Amtospheric chemistry of aldehydes: enhanced peroxyacetyl nitrate formation from ethanol-fueled vehicular emissions. Environ Sci Technol 1988 (22):1026-1034

91 IARC: IARC Monographs on the Evaluation of the Carcinogenic Risk of Chemicals to Humans. Vol. 36. Allylcompounds Aldehydes, Epoxides and Peroxides. International Agency for Research on Cancer, Lyon 1985 pp 101-132

92 IARC: IARC Monographs on the Evaluation of the Carcinogenic Risk of Chemicals to Humans. Vol. 20. Some Halogenated Hydrocarbons. International Agency for Research on Cancer, Lyon 1979 pp 45-545

93 Lane DA, Johnson ND, Barton SC, Thomas GHS, Schroeder WH: Development and evaluation of a novel gas and particle sampler for semi-volatile chlorinated organic compounds in ambient air. Environ Sci Technol 1989 (22):941-947

94 Gregor DJ, Gummer WD: Evidence of atmospheric transport and deposition of organochlorine pesticides and polychlorinated biphenyls in Canadian Arctic snow. Environ Sci Technol 1989 (23):561-565

95 Rapaport RA, Eisenreich SJ: Historical inputs of high molecular weight chlorinated hydrocarbons to Eastern North America. Environ Sci Technol 1988 (22):931-941

96 Duinker C, Bouchertall F: On the distribution of atmospheric polychlorinated biphenyl congeners between vapor phase, aerosol and rain. Environ Sci Technol 1989 (23):57-62

97 Jones KC, Bennett: Human exposure to environmental polychlorinated dibenzo-p-dioxins and dibenzofurans: an exposure committment assessment for 2,3,7,8-TCDD. Sci Total Environ 1989 (78):99-116

98 Erickson MD, Swanson SE, Flura JD, Hinshaw GD: Polychlorinated dibenzofurans and other thermal combustion products from dielectric fluids containing polychlorinated biphenyls. Environ Sci Technol 1989 (23):462-470

99 Rappe C, Bergquist PA, Hansson M: Chemistry and analysis of polychlorinated dioxins and dibenzofurans in biological samples. In Banbury Report 18: Biological Mechanisms of Dioxin Action. NY Cold Springs Harbor Laboratory, Cold Springs Harbor 1984 pp 17-25

100 Hutzinger O, Blumich MJ, Berg Mv, Olie K: Sources and fate of PCDDs and PCDFs: an overview. Chemosphere 1985 (14):551-560

101 Oehme M, Mano S, Mikalsten A, Kerschmer P: Quantitative method for the determination of femtogram amounts of polychlorinated dibenzo-p-dioxins and dibenzofuran as in outdoor air. Chemosphere 1986 (6):455-570

102 Lightowlers PJ, Cape JN: Sources and fate of atmospheric HCl in the U.K. and Western Europe. Atmos Environ 1988 (22):7-15

103 Matthes T: Die Novellierung der Luftstellungnahme zu den fur Abfall Verbrennungsallagen Beatichtigen Aderungen: In: Mullverr-Brennwng 1984, Vortrage der VGB-Konferenz von 28/29 November 1984. Essen FRG. Technische Vereinigung der Grosskraftwerks Betreiber 1984 pp 31-39

104 Molina MJ, Tso TL, Molina LT, Wang FC: Antarctic stratospheric chemistry of chlorine nitrate, hydrogen chloride and ice: release of active chlorine. Science 1987 (238):1253-1257

105 Apsimon HM, Kruse M, Bell JNB: Ammonia emissions and their role in acid deposition. Atmos Environ 1987 (21):1939-1946

106 Asman WAH, Drukker B, Janssen AJ: Modelled historical concentration and depositions of ammonia and ammonium in Europe. Atmos Environ 1988 (22):725-735

107 IARC: IARC Monographs on the Evaluation of Carcinogenic Risk of Chemicals to Man. Vol. 14 Asbestos. International Agency for Research on Cancer, Lyon 1977 p 104

108 WHO: Asbestos and other Natural Mineral Fibres. Environmental Health Criteria No. 53. World Health Organization, Geneva 1986

109 Commins BT: The significance of asbestos and other mineral fibres on environmental ambient air. Commins Assoc, Maidenhead UK, 1985

110 OECD: Air Rept. Env/Air 81.18. 2nd rev. Organization of European Communities Develop, Paris 1984 p 21

111 Nicholson WJ: Asbestos and inorganic fibres. Arbete Och Halsa 1981 (17)

112 IARC: IARC Monographs on the Evaluation of the Carcinogenic Risk of Chemicals to Humans. Vol 42. Silica and Some Silicates. International Agency for Research on Cancer, Lyon 1987

113 Nishioka MG, Howard CC, Contos DA, Ball LM, Lewtas J: Detection of hydroxylated nitro aromatic and hydroxylated nitropolycylic aromatic compound in an ambient air particulate extract using bioassay-directed fractionation. Environ Sci Technol 1988 (22):908-915

114 Lewtas J: Evaluation of the mutagenicity and carcinogenicity of motor vehicle emissions in short term bioassays. Environ Hlth Persp 1983 (47):141-152

115 Stendberg U, Alsberg T, Westerholm R: Emission of carcinogenic components from automobile exhausts. Environ Hlth Persp 1983 (74):53-63

116 Schuetzle D: Sampling of vehicle emissons for chemical analysis and biological testing. Environ Health Persp 1983 (47):65-80

117 Vouk VB, Piver WT: Metallic elements in fossil fuel combustion products: amounts and form of emissions and evaluation of carcinogenicity and mutagenicity. Environ Hlth Persp 1983 (47):201-225

Measurement and Monitoring of Individual Exposures

Kari Hemminki

Institute of Occupational Health, Topeliuksenkatu 41 a A, 00250 Helsinki, Finland

In the previous chapter, the emission sources and levels of air pollutants were surveyed. This chapter will outline strategies for exposure assessment and give exposure estimates.

Humans are exposed to air pollutants in outdoor and indoor air. However, many airborne pollutants are deposited in the course of time and exposure to pollutants may take place not only by inhalation, but also by skin absorption and intake of food and drink (Fig. 1). In general, the physical characteristics of the pollutants (vapour pressure, environmental stability) govern their destination in the ecosystem and determine the route by which humans are exposed. Among the broad classes of pollutants, organic volatiles are primarily taken in by inhalation. By contrast, food is normally the main source of particle-bound persistent chemicals which deposit from the air. Some of these are even enhanced in the food chain. As examples, metals, polycyclic aromatic hydrocarbons and polyhalogenated aromatic compounds are mainly absorbed from food [1]. The focus in this chapter will be on inhalation exposure to airborne carcinogens, while other authors cover other routes of exposure in more detail [2-6]. However, biological exposure monitoring, which will be discussed here, does not distinguish absorption routes for most of the chemicals.

Exposure characteristics change in time and vary from country to country, due to factors such as energy production, traffic intensity, fuels used, cleaning technology in energy production and motor vehicles, construction materials, ventilation systems etc. As a consequence, any exposure estimate should be treated with caution.

Exposure Assessment Strategies

The analytical techniques for most chemical classes have improved enormously during the past few decades. A dramatic illustration of this is seen for dioxins such as 2,3,7,8-TCDD, whose detection limit in environmental samples was about 1,000,000 pg/g in 1965; 20 years later it was 0.001 pg/g [7]. Similarly, the precision of the methods has improved: while one chromatographic peak contained up to 20 possible dioxin isomers in 1965, today single isomers are separated [7]. Obviously, the advances in analytical chemistry exceed by far the advances in toxicology of the pollutants. A word of caution is due concerning the measurement of any complex

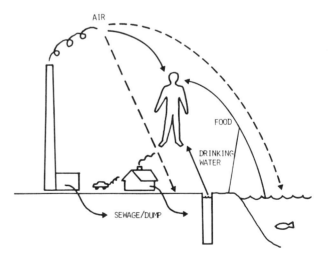

Fig. 1. Sources of human exposure to environmental contaminants. Broken lines indicate deposition to water and soil

samples in previous decades: the results may be unreliable.

Exposure to individual chemicals may be estimated by stationary samplers, personal samplers, or from exhaled air. Also blood and urine samples are used, as mentioned in the section on biological monitoring. Measurements from exhaled air are usually considered part of biological monitoring, but here they will be discussed in the context of ambient air monitoring.

Ambient Air Monitoring

The US Environmental Protection Agency has sponsored a comprehensive study, the "Total Exposure Assessment Methodology (TEAM) Study" [5], which addresses many important issues regarding the analysis of organic volatile compounds. I will quote some examples from this study, and recommend anyone working in the field to consult the primary source for further details.

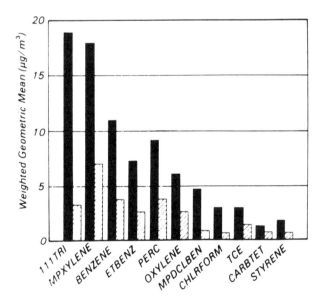

Fig. 2. Estimated geometric mean values of 11 toxic compounds in daytime (6:00 am - 6:00 pm) air samples for the population of Elizabeth and Bayonne, New Jersey, USA, between September and November 1981. Personal air estimates (black bars) based on 340 samples; outdoor air estimates (hatched bars) based on 88 samples. Reproduced with permission from ref. 5

Levels of pollutants differ by season and by the hour of day, depending on the source of emission. For most of the volatile organic chemicals measured in the TEAM study, the indoor concentrations exceeded the outdoor concentrations (about 2-fold), and when clear indoor sources of emission existed, the non-occupational indoor concentrations were much (sometimes up to 100 times) higher [5]. This was seen in many other studies as well [8-15]. Some of the main contributors to indoor emissions of organic material include smoking, burning, cooking, building materials, furniture cleaners, moth crystals, hot showers and printed materials.

As regards particulate exposures, indoor concentrations may be lower than outdoor concentrations because some filtration may take place. Of course, indoor particulate emissions also exists, sources being smoking, burning of wood or coal, cooking, etc.

Personal monitoring with adequate population sampling gives a more accurate estimate of individual human exposures than stationary monitors. In the TEAM study, exhaled air samples correlated highly with personal monitors. However, exhaled air samples give lower exposure estimates than personal monitors, possibly because of distribution, metabolism and deposition of the chemical in the body.

Personal monitoring is also important because it shows in which type of environment humans spend their time. Although many studies have shown that people living in the Western countries spend a vast proportion of their time indoors, mainly at home or in the workplace, most air monitoring is carried out outdoors.

The indoor and outdoor concentrations of most volatile organics differ only marginally for many compounds, but personal monitoring shows larger differences because much more time is spent indoors than outdoors. Figure 2 shows results from the TEAM study for 11 chemicals measured in the daytime outdoors and by personal samplers for New Jersey residents. Personal monitoring shows 2 to 5 times higher exposure than outdoor measurements would give.

Personal monitoring would be even more important for particulate than gaseous compounds because diffusion of particulate material is limited as compared to gases.

Table 1. Population quantiles by respirable size particle (RSP) concentrations [16]

Sampling	(N)	RSP Quantile μg/m³					
		95%	75%	50%	25%	5%	Mean
Personal	(249)	113.0	48.5	34.0	25.5	17.0	43.9
Indoor	(266)	118.6	46.0	29.0	20.0	10.0	41.6
Outdoor	(71)	33.4	23.0	17.0	13.0	7.2	18.0

Unfortunately, limited data is available for particle-bound compounds. In one study, respirable particles were measured by personal samplers and stationary samplers located outdoors and indoors in a room used most frequently (Table 1). Personal samplers produced the highest values, but only slightly above the indoor monitor. The outdoor levels were about 40% of the indoor levels [16,17]. This probably implied the existence of indoor sources of particulate material.

A salient finding in the TEAM study was a wide variation in exposure among individuals. The ranges were 1,000 or even 10,000-fold. However, if the population was truncated by deleting 10% from both extremes, the range in exposure was about 10 to 20-fold. Figure 3 illustrates the exposure of various fractions of the population to benzene, but the distribution of exposure to other volatile organics is quite similar. These data clearly convey that references to "average", "mean" or "median" exposure must be taken with caution, but such summary classifications have to be used for simplicity or lack of data.

Biological Monitoring

Biological monitoring refers to measurement of chemicals or their metabolites in biological samples such as blood or urine. Biological monitoring has a long tradition in occupational health, and for many compounds it is part of a routine surveillance activity. For a number of chemicals, equations have been derived which relate ambient air levels of chemicals to their concentrations in biological samples.

Measurements of environmental pollutants have been taken from biological samples, particularly in those cases where inhalation exposure is not the only, nor the principal source of exposure [18,19]; for example, measurements of metals such as lead and

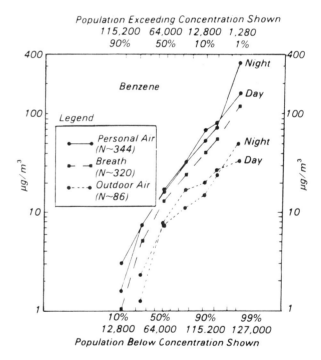

Fig. 3. Estimated frequency distributions of personal air exposures, outdoor air concentrations, and exhaled breath values of benzene for the Elizabeth-Bayonne population. All air values are 12-hour integrated samples. The breath value was taken following the daytime air sample (6:00 am - 6:00 pm). All outdoor air samples were taken in the vicinity of the participants' homes. Reproduced with permission from ref. 5

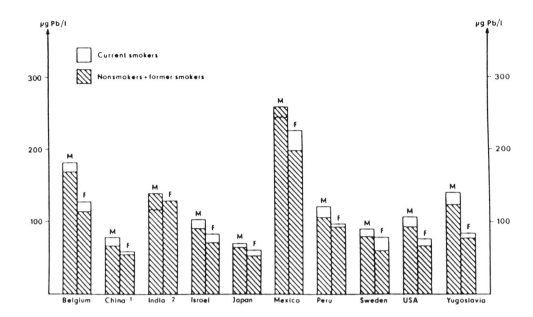

Fig. 4. Concentrations of lead in blood (median values) for male (M) and female (F) teachers, subdivided into smokers and nonsmokers (including former smokers). Indian data represent teachers in Ahmedabad. Swedish data represent a random sample of the total population in Stockholm. 1) only 2 female smokers; 2) no female smokers.
Reproduced with permission from ref. 18

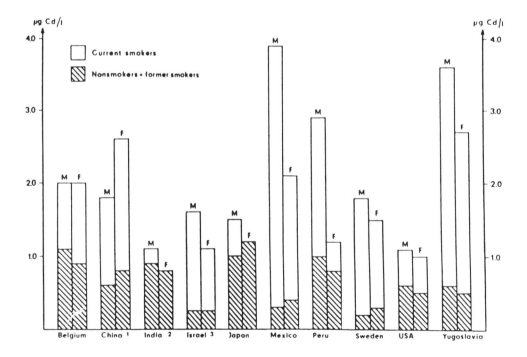

Fig. 5. Concentrations of cadmium in blood (median values) for male (M) and female (F) teachers, subdivided into smokers and nonsmokers (including former smokers). Indian data represent teachers in Ahmedabad. Swedish data represent a random sample of the total population in Stockholm. 1) Only 2 female smokers; 2) no female smokers; 3) the values for nonsmokers are given as 0.25 µg Cd/l, i.e., half the detection limit. Reproduced with permission from ref. 18

Table 2. Protein-binding levels and interindividual variation in humans

Exposure	Level (μg/g)	Interindividual variation noted	Reference
Cisplatin, haemoglobin	1-3	3-5	23
Cisplatin, plasma protein	10-50	2-2.5	23
Smoking, hydroxyethyl-valine in haemoglobin	~0.05	3-4	24
Smoking, 4-aminobiphenyl in haemoglobin	0.00015	3	27
Background, hydroxyethyl-valine in haemoglobin	0.008	2.5-5	24-26
Background, 4-aminobiphenyl in haemoglobin	0.00003	6	27

cadmium, which are mainly obtained by ingestion of polluted food. Their origin is, therefore, air pollution (see Chapter 2). An international comparison was made between teachers who were not subject to occupational exposure to these compounds (Figs. 4 and 5) [18]. According to the Finnish Institute of Occupational Health, lead and cadmium levels are below 200 μg/l and 1.1 μg/l (non-smokers), respectively, in non-exposed individuals. The teachers in Mexico exceed these values for lead; non-smoking teachers in Belgium and Japan are just at that level for cadmium. The marked effect of smoking on the cadmium levels is clearly seen in Figure 5.

A new area in biological monitoring is the measurement of protein- and DNA-binding products of the compounds that are capable of reacting covalently with macromolecules, a property shared by many carcinogens [20,21]. DNA-adducts, mechanistically related to the initiation events of cancer, give a measure of the target dose. However, in most cases true target tissues cannot be obtained and therefore surrogate tissues, such as white blood cells, are being used. Protein binding is usually measured from haemoglobin or plasma protein [22]. Table 2 lists the protein-binding studies where exposure levels have been quantitated in humans. Similarly, DNA-binding studies are listed in Table 3; the tissues analysed were in most cases white blood

cells or lymphocytes [21,28]. Protein- and DNA-binding studies have also been carried out in the occupational environment and estimated exposures appear to be correlated with the level of adducts [21,28]. Some types of adducts can be detected in all individuals, either through environmental exposure or endogenous adduct formation.

In 2 studies, attempts were made to assess the contribution of environmental pollution to the level of macromolecular adducts. In one study carried out in Sweden, 2-hydroxyethyl adducts (produced by ethylene oxide, a metabolite of ethene), were determined in N-terminal valines of haemoglobin from groups of urban and rural inhabitants [25]. No difference was found. In another study, Silesian urban areas were compared to unpolluted Polish countryside by assaying for aromatic adducts in white blood cell DNA by ^{32}p-post-labelling and immunoassay [39]. Individuals from the urban area displayed about 3 times as many adducts as the population from the rural area. The adduct patterns resembled those obtained from Silesian coke workers, suggesting that derivates of coal burning and extraction may contribute to the finding. Some evidence of pollution-related cancer risk has been obtained in the Cracow area of Poland (see Chapter 5).

Cytogenetic studies where chromosomal aberrations, sister chromatid exchanges and micronuclei are measured, have been used

Table 3. DNA-binding levels and interindividual variation reported in human tissues

Exposure/system (tissue)	Level (adduct/10^8 nucleotides)	Interindividual variation noted	Reference
Cisplatin (WBC)	~50	1.5 (15)[1]	29
Smoking, aromatic postlabelling (Lung)	1-30	5-10	30
Smoking, aromatic PAH postlabelling and immunoassay (WBC)	1-30	10	31-33
Foundries, cokeries postlabelling and immunoassay (WBC)	1-1000	100	34-40
Background, aromatic (WBC)	1-10	2-20	28

1   one individual; WBC = white blood cells

to monitor the effects of exposure to chemicals. The main application has been in occupational monitoring, where for several carcinogenic exposures elevations of one or several of the cytogenetic parameters have been noted [41,42]. The assays measure genetic damage inflicted by exposure and they are particularly useful in the case of complex, poorly identified exposures.

Exposure to Carcinogens Outdoors

For a detailed discussion of the levels and sources of outdoor air pollutants, the reader is referred to Chapter 2 of this volume.

Inorganic Particles

Metals are bound to particles in outdoor air, and their concentrations depend on the proximity to the sources. Industrial emissions and waste incineration are the main sources of most carcinogenic metals in the atmosphere, although the main source of lead is lead-containing petrol. Outdoor air is usually a minor (direct) source of exposure to metals: food and, for arsenic and cadmium, smoking are the main sources [1,6]. However, many metals, such as lead and cadmium [1], are absorbed to a higher degree when inhaled than when ingested, indicating the health significance of exposure by inhalation.

For arsenic, the representative background levels are 1-10 ng/m^3 in rural areas; urban concentrations may exceed 100 ng/m^3. Communities with nonferrous metal smelters and power plants may have air concentrations of micrograms per cubic metre. The concentration of cadmium in rural areas is in the order of 0.1-5 ng/m^3; in urban areas the concentration ranges between 5 and 15 ng/m^3 and is even higher in communities with cadmium-emitting industrial sources [1].

The carcinogenic effects of the various chromium compounds vary with the valency state, among other factors, hexavalent chromium compounds being the demonstrated carcinogenic species [1]. The chromium compounds commonly found in nature are mainly trivalent, as are the species found in air particles. Measured as chromium, rural air concentrations range between 0.1 and 1 ng/m^3, as compared to urban concentrations of 1-100 ng/m^3. For lead compounds, rural air concentrations are in the range of 0.1-0.3 µg/m^3, while those in urban areas go up to 3 µg/m^3 in Europe. The concentrations of nickel range between 0.1-1 ng/m^3 in rural and 1-100 ng/m^3 in urban areas [1].

Asbestiform fibres in air are another potential source of carcinogens. Emissions into the atmosphere come mainly from man-made sources, such as refining and construction, brake linings and disposal. The air levels are thought to be generally below 100 fibres/m^3 in rural areas and below 1,000 fibres/m^3 in urban areas.

Particulate Organic Material

Soot particles contain PAHs which are formed as a result of pyrolytic processes, especially incomplete combustion of organic materials. A number of heterocyclic aromatic compounds (e.g., carbazole, acridine) as well as PAH with one or several NO_2 groups (nitro-PAH) can also be generated by incomplete combustion. Nitro-PAHs are readily formed from PAHs through a nitration reaction and they are present in most environmental samples were PAHs are found, but in lesser quantities [43-45].
The natural background level of benzo(a)pyrene (not including that from forest fires and volcanic eruptions) may be almost zero. In the 1970s in the USA, the annual average level of benzo(a)pyrene in urban areas without coke ovens was less than 1

ng/m^3 and that in other cities 1-5 ng/m^3. In the 1960s, the annual average values in several European cities were above 100 ng/m^3.

Volatile Organic Carcinogens

Representative measurements of outdoor air concentrations of organic volatile compounds were carried out in the TEAM study [3]. Table 4 summarises results of measurements made in urban areas of New Jersey and California (USA) during various seasons. Among the compounds listed, the median concentrations are highest for benzene (1.7-1.9 µg/m^3). The concentrations of ortho-, meta- and para-xylene and ethylbenzene, which have not been shown to be carcinogenic, approximate those of benzene (data not shown). The other listed compounds were present at up to microgram per cubic metre levels. The range of concentrations given covers about one order of magnitude, the lowest concentrations being found in small urban centres.
Formaldehyde was not measured, but I have included it in Table 4 for the sake of later comparisons. According to the World Health Organisation, the natural background level is a few micrograms per cubic metre, and concentrations in urban air are about 5-10 µg/m^3.

Table 4. Volatile organic carcinogens in overnight outdoor air samples in US urban areas (New Jersey and California, 1981-84) [5]

Volatile organic carcinogen	Median concentration (µg/m^3)	90th percentile (µg/m^3)
Benzene	1.7 - 19	3.2 - 32
Carbon tetrachloride	0.33 - 0.81	0.47 - 2.5
Chloroform	0.03 - 0.66	0.06 - 44
Meta, para, dichlorobenzene	0.25 - 1.7	1.0 - 5.9
1,4-Dioxane	0.02 - 0.26	0.53 - 1.4
Formaldehyde [1]	1 - 10	
Styrene	0.23 - 4.2	1.0 - 8.3
Tetrachloroethylene	0.25 - 7.4	0.61 - 24

1   From World Health Organisation [1]; annual average concentrations in urban air

Ethylene and propylene are precursors (about 5% conversion in the human body) of ethylene oxide and propylene oxide, both shown to cause cancer in experimental animals. Ethylene is present at levels of 10-20 $\mu g/m^3$ and propylene of 1-10 $\mu g/m^3$ in urban air [25].

Radon

Radon-222 is a member of the radioactive decay chain of uranium-238, and radon-220 (often referred to as thoron) is a member of the decay chain of thorium-232. The half-life of radon-222 is 3.8 days, and it decays into short-lived isotopes of polonium, lead, bismuth and thallium, which are referred to as radon daughters. In closed spaces, radon and its daughters are in equilibrium: for one unit of radon there are 0.3-0.5 units of its daughters [46,47]. Uranium and radium occur abundantly in the earth's crust. The average concentration of radon gas in the atmosphere at ground level is about 3 Bq/m^3, with a range of 0.1 (over oceans) to 10 Bq/m^3 (1 Bq=27 pCi). The concentration of radon varies widely in different parts of the world. High concentrations of radon have been noted especially in areas where terrestrial gamma radiation is high. Radon and its daughters are usually present in a particle-bound form.

Exposure to Carcinogens Indoors

Few data are available on the concentration of particle-bound carcinogens such as metals, asbestiform fibres and PAHs in indoor air. The concentration of asbestos is thought to be no higher indoors than it is outdoors (e.g., below 1,000 fibres/m^3), unless it was used as coating material [1]. When asbestos was used in indoor or ventilation coatings, concentrations of up to 10,000 fibres/m^3 have been measured. In the Cappadocian region in Turkey, erionite-containing rock has been used traditionally as building and insulation material, and indoor air samples in such constructions also contain up to 10,000 fibres/m^3. In Cappadocian villages, even outdoor fibre concentrations may be as high as 3,000 fibres/m^3 [48].

The levels of PAHs in indoor air depend on the types of combustion and fuel as well as the ventilation and exhaust systems used. When no proper chimneys are present, indoor concentrations may reach very high levels [1]. Even wood-burning stoves and fireplaces tend to result in some leakage of PAHs into indoor air [49-52]. In non-occupational environments, indoor and outdoor air are thought to be minor (direct) sources of exposure to PAHs, and food is the main source [1].

Table 5. Volatile organic carcinogens in overnight indoor air samples in US homes in urban areas (New Jersey and California, 1981-1984) [5]

Volatile organic carcinogen	Median concentration ($\mu g/m^3$)	90th percentile ($\mu g/m^3$)
Benzene	4.4 - 15	16 - 30
Carbon tetrachloride	0.65 - 1.5	0.9 - 5.8
Chloroform	0.03 - 3.3	2.4 - 16
Meta, para, dichlorobenzene	0.53 - 4.2	8.4 - 140
1,4-Dioxane	0.03 - 0.24	0.36 - 3.0
Formaldehyde [1]	50 - 200	
Styrene	0.71 - 28	2.0 - 6.7
Tetrachloroethylene	1.8 - 8.3	4.2 - 36

1   From World Health Organisation [1], for conventional buildings not containing large amounts of particle board

Volatile organic chemicals have been measured in indoor air in the study of the US Environmental Protection Agency [5], in residences in New Jersey and California (Table 5) in the same areas as the outdoor measurements shown in Table 4. The indoor concentrations of all the listed compounds exceeded the outdoor concentrations. Such differences have been seen in many other studies [5], which shows the importance of indoor sources of these chemicals, including building materials, paints, glues, furnishings, dry-cleaned clothes, cigarettes, petrol, cleansers, moth crystals, hot showers and printed materials [5].

Formaldehyde was not measured in the above study, but many other studies are available [1]. Average indoor air concentrations are 0.05-0.2 mg/m^3 (Table 5); in trailers and new houses, with ample use of (low-grade) particle board, concentrations may reach 1 mg/m^3. The indoor concentrations of formaldehyde exceed those outside by almost 2 orders of magnitude.

Environmental tobacco smoke consists of sidestream smoke and exhaled mainstream smoke. The sidestream smoke is formed at lower temperatures and at different oxygen levels than the mainstream smoke. Some 10% (400) of the individual compounds in tobacco smoke have been identified so far in the sidestream smoke [53]. In non-filter cigarettes, the sidestream smoke contains greater amounts of many compounds, such as nitrosamines and aromatic amines, than the mainstream smoke [53]. The sidestream smoke of filter cigarettes is thought to be similar in composition to that of non-filter cigarettes [53]. Many types of tobacco-related pollutants have been measured in spaces where people smoke [5,53]. The concentration of nitrosamines and polycyclic aromatic hydrocarbons exceeded those found in polluted urban air by 1 to 3 orders of magnitude.

Of all the environmental carcinogens, radon and its daughters belong to the most important ones. There are 3 indoor sources: the ground, building materials and water. The potential for entry from the ground depends mainly on the concentration of radium in the soil and on the permeability of the soil to radon. For people who live close to the ground, e.g., in detached houses or on the ground floor of multi-family buildings without cellars, the most important source of radon is thought to be the ground [1,54,55]. Another potential source of radon is building materials. The emanation of radon from construction materials depends not only on the radium concentration but also on factors such as the fraction of radon released from the material, the porosity of the material and the surface and finish used. Building materials containing gypsum and concrete containing alum shale may have high radium concentrations. The concentrations of radon in brick and concrete may also be high if the raw materials were taken from locations with high levels of natural radioactivity [1,54,55]. Radon also diffuses into underground water reservoirs, and exposure may occur when the water is used. In wells drilled into rock, radium and radon concentrations in the water may be high. When this water is used in households, radon is released into indoor air and causes an increase in the average radon concentration. Usually, radon daughters release into air result in higher exposures than radon daughters that remain in drinking water; however, parent radium-226 remaining in water occurs at 0.1 Bq/l in water from wells drilled in rock of high radium content, as in Maine and Iowa (USA), Scandinavia and Finland [1].

In Europe and North America, the mean radon daughter concentrations range between 10 and 50 Bq/m^3, with the highest averages reported in Scandinavia [1]. A small fraction of dwellings, approximately 1%, have concentrations more than 10 times higher than the national average [1]. Importantly, due to better insulation and lower ventilation, radon levels indoors have been increasing lately.

Summary of Exposure Levels

The exposures discussed above are summarised in Table 6. The method of obtaining the values is an approximation of the measured levels discussed earlier in this chapter. As the people in industrialised countries spend most of their time indoors, the estimates were weighed towards indoor levels, if no personal sampling data were available.

Table 6. Estimated concentrations of airborne carcinogens or their precursors in urban and rural areas of industrialised countries such as Finland

Compound	Urban areas[1] ($\mu g/m^3$)	Rural areas[1] ($\mu g/m^3$)
Arsenic[2]	0.1	0.001
Cadmium[2]	0.01	0.001
Chromium[2]	0.01	0.001
Lead[2]	3	0.1
Nickel[2]	0.01	0.001
Asbestos (fibers/m^3)[2,3]	<1000	<100
Benzene	10	1
Benzo(a)pyrene [4,5]	0.01	0.01
Carbon tetrachloride	1	0.1
Chloroform	1	0.1
Dichlorobenzenes	1	0.1
1,4-Dioxane	0.1	0.01
Ethene	10	1
Formaldehyde[5]	100	20
Propene	5	0.5
Radon (Bq/m^3)[5]	20	40
Styrene	1	0.1
Tetrachloroethylene	5	0.5

1   The figures have been rounded, see text
2   No representative indoor measurement available
3   If asbestos was used in insulation and coatings, the concentrations may be much higher
4   Assuming some wood or coal burning at homes
5   The estimate is based on indoor concentrations

Representative indoor measurements are not available for particle-bound carcinogens such as metals. Therefore, the outdoor levels were used for both urban and rural areas. Although the air levels of asbestos may be quite low, particularly in rural areas, use of asbestos in insulation or coating may cause drastic increases in exposure. At present, there is no way to consider such factors in the population exposure estimates. Environmental tobacco smoke is an important environmental carcinogen, but individual life-style factors, rather than the urban-rural difference, are crucial for exposure.

For the volatile organic carcinogens, mainly the TEAM data were used in the exposure estimates. Usually, the rural levels were considered to be lower by a factor of 10. The outdoor levels of most pollutants are likely to be less than 10% in rural areas as compared to urban areas, but as the indoor exposures are usually prevailing, 10% was considered a compromising figure. As regards radon exposure, rural areas were thought to be affected more because of ground-level, single-family housing. Measurements from Finland clearly point in this direction. This is likely to be an important confounding factor in epidemiological studies, because radon is a very important environmental carcinogen [1,6].

Natural gas and propane may contain rather large amounts of radon. However, exposure to it will occur, in most cases, at much lower levels because of the loss of radioactivity during gas distribution. The only instance where there might be a potentially significant exposure to radon indoors is when a great deal of gas is burnt without adequate exhaust of the fuels [56].

With all these qualifications and reservations, it appears that, by and large, the urban population is exposed to many carcinogens at levels of about 10 times higher than the rural population. The exceptions may be radon, as explained above, and benzo(a)pyrene and other polycyclic aromatic hydrocarbons, assuming that more individual heating and wood burning takes place in rural areas. For formaldehyde, the difference was estimated to be 5-fold only because of a lesser use of formaldehyde-emitting building materials and higher ventilation rates in rural homes.

Acknowledgements

I wish to thank the members of the Task Force whose comments were duly incorporated in the text.

REFERENCES

1   World Health Organization: Air Quality Guidelines for Europe. World Health Organization, Copenhagen 1987

2   Hemminki K, Vainio H, Sorsa M, Salminen S: An estimation of the exposure of the population in Finland to suspected chemical carcinogens. Environ Carcinogen Rev Cl 1983:55-95

3   Hemminki K, Vainio H: Human exposure to potentially carcinogenic compounds. In: Berlin A, Draper M, Hemminki K and Vainio H (eds) Monitoring Human Exposure to Carcinogenic and Mutagenic Agents. IARC Scientific Publications. IARC, Lyon 1984 (59) 37-45

4   International Agency for Research on Cancer. IARC Monographs on the Evaluation of Carcinogenc Risks to Humans. Suppl 7: Overall Evaluations of Carcinogenicity: An Updating of IARC Monographs. IARC, Lyon 1987 pp 1-42

5   Environmental Protection Agency: The Total Exposure Assessment Methodology (TEAM) Study: Summary and Analysis. US Environmental Protection Agency, Washington DC 1987 pp 1-3

6   Hemminki K: Environmental carcinogens. In: Cooper CS, Grover PL (eds) Handbook of Experimental Pharmacology. Springer Verlag, Heidelberg 1989 pp 31-61

7   Crummett WB, Nestrick RJ, Lamparski LL: Analytical methodology for the determination of PCDDs in environmental samples: an overview and critique. In: Kamrin MA, Rodgers PW (eds) Dioxins in the Environment. Hemisphere Publ Co, Washington DC 1985 pp 57-83

8   Mølhave L, Moller J: The atmospheric environment in modern Danish dwellings: measurements in 39 flats. In: Indoor Climate, Danish Building Research Institute, Copenhagen 1979 pp 171-186

9   Jarke FH, Gordon S, Dravnieks A: ASHRAE Report #87. IITRI, Chicago 1981

10   Lebret E, Van de Wiel HJ, Bos HP, Noij D, Boleij JSM: Volatile hydrocarbons in Dutch homes. In: Indoor Air, Swedish Council for Building Research, Stockholm 1984 (4):169-174

11   Seifert B, Abraham HJ: Indoor air concentrations of benzene and some other aromatic hydrocarbons. Ecotoxicol Environ Safety 1982 (6):190-192

12   De Bortoli M, Knoppel H, Pecchio E, Peil A, Rogora L, Schauenberg H, Schlitt H, Vissers H: Integrating real life measurements of organic pollution in indoor and outdoor air of homes in northern Italy. In: Indoor Air, Swedish Council for Building Research, Stockholm 1984 (4):21-26

13   Gammage RB, White DA, Gupta KC: Residential measurements of high volatility organics and their sources. In: Indoor Air, Swedish Council for Building Research, Stockholm 1984 (4):157-162

14   Monteith KD, Stock TH, Seifert WE Jr: Sources and characterization of organic air contaminants inside manufactured housing. In: Indoor Air, Swedish Council for Building Research, Stockholm 1984 (4):285-290

15   Girman JR, Hodgson AT, Newton AS: Volatile organic emissions from adhesives with indoor applications. In: Indoor Air, Swedish Council for Building Research, Stockholm 1984 (4):271-276

16   Mage DT: Concepts of human exposure assessment for airborne particulate matter. Environ Int 1985 (11):407-412

17   van Houdt JJ: Indoor and outdoor airborne particles: an in vitro study on mutagenic potentials and toxicological implications. Thesis at Wageningen Agricultural University, Wageningen, The Netherlands 1988 pp

18   Vahter M: Assessment of Human Exposure to Lead and Cadmium Through Biological Monitoring. National Swedish Institute of Environmental Medicine, Stockholm 1982

19   Slorach SA, Vaz R: PCB levels in breast milk: data from the UNCP/WHO pilot project on biological monitoring and some other recent studies. Environ Health Perspect 1985 (60):121-126

20   Weinstein IB: The origins of human cancer: molecular mechanisms of carcinogenesis and their implications for cancer prevention and treatment. Cancer Res 1988 (48):4135-4143

21   Bartsch H, Hemminki K, O'Neill IK: Methods for Detecting DNA Damaging Agents in Humans: Applications in Cancer Epidemiology and Prevention. International Agency for Research on Cancer, Lyon, IARC Scientific Publication 1988 (89)

22   Neumann HG: Analysis of hemoglobin as a dose monitor for alkylating and arylating agents. Arch Toxicol 1984 (56):1-6

23   Mustonen R, Hietanen P, Leppälä S, Takala M, Hemminki K: Determination of cis-diamminedichloroplatinum (II) in plasma proteins and hemoglobin of cancer patients. Arch Toxicol 1989 (63):361-366

24   Törnqvist M, Österman-Golkar S, Kautiainen A, Jensen S, Farmer PB, Ehrenberg L: Tissue doses of ethylene oxide in cigarette smokers determined from adduct levels in hemoglobin. Carcinogenesis 1986 (7):1519-1521

25   Törnqvist M: Monitoring and Cancer Risk Assessment of Carcinogens Particularly Alkenes in Urban Air. Doctoral Thesis, University of Stockholm 1989

26   Bailey E, Brooks AGF, Dollery CT, Farmer PB, Passingham BJ, Sleightholm MA, Yates DW: Hydroxyethylvaline adduct formation in haemoglobin as a biological monitor of cigarette smoke intake. Arch Toxicol 1988 (62):247-253

27   Bryant MS, Skipper PL, Tannenbaum SR, Maclure M: Hemoglobin adducts of 4-aminobiphelyl in smokers and nonsmokers. Cancer Res 1987 (47):602-608

28   Perera F, Mayer J, Santella RM, Brenner D, Jeffrey A, Latriano L, Smith S, Warburton D, Young TL, Tsai WY, Hemminki K, Brandt-Rauf P: Biologic markers in risk assessment for environmental carcinogens. Environ Health Persp 1989 (in press)

29   Fichtinger-Schepman AMJ, van Oosterom AT, Lohman PHM, Berends F: Cis-diamminedichloroplatinum (II)-induced DNA adducts in peripheral leukocytes from seven cancer patients: quantitative immunological detection of the adduct induction and removal after a single dose of

cis-diamminedichloroplatinum (II). Cancer Res 1987 (47):3000-3004

30 Phillips DH, Hewer A, Martin CN, Garner RC, King MM: Correlation of DNA adduct levels in human lung with cigarette smoking. Nature 1988 (336):790-792

31 Everson RB, Randerath E, Santella RM, Cefalo RC, Avitts TA, Randerath K: Detection of smoking-related covalent DNA adducts in human placenta. Science 1986 (231):54-57

32 Randerath E, Miller RH, Mittal D, Avitts TA, Dunsford HA, Randerath K: Covalent DNA damage in tissues of cigarette smokers as determined by ^{32}p-postlabelling assay. JNCI 1989 (81):341-347

33 Perera FP, Santella RM, Brenner D, Poirier MC, Munshi AA, Fischman HK, Ryzin JV: DNA adducts, protein adducts and sister chromatid exchange in cigarette smokers and nonsmokers. JNCI 1987 (79):449-456

34 Weston A, Rowe RM, Manchester DK, Farmer PB, Mann DL, Harris CC: Fluorescence and mass spectral evidence for the formation of benzo(a)pyrene anti-diol-epoxine-DNA and hemoglobin adducts in humans. Carcinogenesis 1989 (10):251-257

35 Perera FP, Hemminki K, Young TL, Santella RM, Brenner D, Kelly G: Detection of polycyclic aromatic hydrocarbon-DNA adducts in white blood cells of foundry workers. Cancer Res 1988 (48):2288-2291

36 Shamsuddin AKM, Sinopoli NT, Hemminki K, Boesch RR, Harris CC: Detection of benzo(a)pyrene: DNA adducts in human white blood cells. Cancer Res 1985 (45):66-68

37 Harris CC, Vähäkangas K, Newman MJ, Trivers GE, Shamsuddin A, Sinopoli N, Mann DL, Wright WE: Detection of benzo(a)pyrene diol epoxide-DNA adducts in peripheral blood lymphocytes and antibodies to the adducts in serum from coke oven workers. Proc Nat Acad Sciences USA 1985 (82):6672-6676

38 Haugen A, Becher G, Benestad C, Vähäkangas K, Trivers GE, Newman MJ, Harris CC: Determination of polycyclic aromatic hydrocarbons in the urine, benzo(a)pyrene diol epoxide-DNA adducts in lymphocyte DNA, and antibodies to the adducts in sera from coke oven workers exposed to measured amounts of polycyclic aromatic hydrocarbons in the work atmosphere. Cancer Res 1986 (46):4178-4183

39 Hemminki K, Grzybowska E, Chorazy M, Twardowska-Saucha K, Sroczynski JW, Putman KL, Randerath K, Phillips DH, Hewer A, Santella RM, Perera FP: DNA adducts in humans related to occupational and environmental exposure to aromatic compounds. IARC Scientific Publications (in press)

40 Phillips DH, Hemminki K, Alhonen A, Hewer A, Grover PL: Monitoring occupational exposure to carcinogens: detection by ^{32}p-postlabelling of aromatic DNA adducts in white blood cells from iron foundry workers. Mutation Res 1988 (204):531-541

41 Vainio H, Sorsa M, Hemminki K: Biological monitoring in surveillance of exposure to genotoxicants. Am J Industr Med 1983 (4):87-103

42 Sorsa M: Genotoxicology. In: Zenz C (ed) Occupational Medicine. Year Book Med Publishers, Chicago, London, Boca Ration 1988 (2):806-814

43 Rosenkranz HS, Mermelstein R: The genotoxicity, metabolism and carcinogenicity of nitrated polycyclic aromatic hydrocarbons. J Environ Sci Health 1985 (3C):221-272

44 White CM: Analysis of nitrated polycyclic aromatic hydrocarbons by gas chromatography. In: White CM (ed) Nitrated Polycyclic Aromatic Hydrocarbons. A Hüthig Verlag, Heidelberg 1985 pp 1-86

45 International Agency for Research on Cancer. IARC Monographs on the Evaluation of Carcinogenic Risks to Humans. IARC, Lyon 1989 (46)

46 UNSCEAR. Report to the General Assembly with Annexes. Ionizing Radiation: Sources and Biological Effects. United Nations: New York 1982

47 International Agency for Research on Cancer. IARC Monographs on the Evaluation of Carcinogenic Risks to Humans. IARC, Lyon 1988 (43)

48 International Agency for Research on Cancer. IARC Monographs on the Evaluation of Carcinogenic Risk of Chemicals to Humans. IARC, Lyon 1987 (42)

49 Häsänen E, Pohjola V, Pyysalo H et al: Polycyclic aromatic hydrocarbons in Finnish sauna air. Sci Total Environ 1984 (37):223-231

50 Alfheim I, Becher G, Hongslo JK, Lazaridis G, Löfroth G, Rahmdahl T, Rivedal E, Salomaa S, Sanner T and Sorsa M: Short-term bioassays of fractionated emission samples from wood combustion. Teratog Carcinog Mutagen 1984 (4):459-475

51 Alfheim I, Becher G, Hongslo JK and Rahmdahl T: Mutagenicity testing of high performance liquid chromatography fractions from wood stove emission samples using a modified Salmonella assay requiring smaller sampling volumes. Environ Mutagen 1984 (6):91-102

52 Alink GM, Smit HA, van Houdt JJ, Kolkman JR and Boley JSM: Mutagenic activity of airborne particulates at non-industrial locations. Mutation Res 1983 (116):21-34

53 International Agency for Research on Cancer. IARC Monographs on the Evaluation of Carcinogenic Risks to Humans. IARC, Lyon 1985 (38)

54 Mossman KL, Thomas DS, Dritschilo A: Environmental radiation and cancer. Environ Carinog Rev 1986 (C4, 2):119-161

55 Velema JP: Contaminated drinking water as a potential cause of cancer in humans. Environ Carcinog Rev 1987 (C5):1-28

56 Bruno RC: Sources of indoor radon in houses: A review. J Air Pollution Control Assoc 1983 (33):105-109

Experimental Evidence for the Carcinogenicity of Air Pollutants

Joellen Lewtas

Health Effects Research Laboratory, U.S. Environmental Protection Agency, Research Triangle Park, NC 27711, U.S.A.

The role of air pollution in human lung cancer has been difficult to assess or quantitate due to the many confounding exposures and factors that influence human cancer (see Chapter 5). This is especially true for cancers of the respiratory tract where the vast majority of cancers have been related to cigarette smoking. Much of our understanding of the potential human risk from air pollution is derived from experimental cancer studies on both individual chemicals and mixtures of air pollutants [1]. This chapter discusses the experimental evidence for the carcinogenicity of air pollutants in long-term animal cancer studies and from short-term bioassays. The evidence is organised and discussed in 3 categories of exposures: (a) individual chemicals found as air pollutants (e.g., formaldehyde); (b) mixtures emitted from air pollution sources (e.g., automotive emissions); and (c) mixtures of air pollution taken from ambient air (e.g., urban air particulate matter).

Although definitive evidence of carcinogenicity in humans can be provided only by human epidemiological and clinical studies, experimental studies in animals and short-term bioassays provide evidence that is considered relevant to the classification and prediction of potential human cancer risk [2]. This chapter will consider the following 2 types of experimental evidence for carcinogenicity of air pollutants: animal cancer bioassays, which are generally considered to be long-term tests, and short-term bioassays for genetic and related effects.

Animal Cancer Bioassays

A high proportion of the chemicals or mixtures which are known from epidemiological studies to be carcinogenic to humans and which are suitable for a long-term animal cancer bioassay, have been shown to induce cancer in animals in at least one species through experimental methods [3,4]. The fraction of animal carcinogens which are also human carcinogens is unknown. The International Agency for Research on Cancer (IARC) [2] has stated in its *Monographs on the Evaluation of Carcinogenic Risks to Humans*, the view that is also held by many other international and national health organisations, namely that "...in the absence of adequate data on humans, it is biologically plausible and prudent to regard agents and mixtures for which there is sufficient evidence of carcinogenicity in experimental animals as if they presented a carcinogenic risk to humans..." [2].

The evidence relevant to carcinogenicity in experimental animals is classified by IARC into one of the following categories:

(a) *Sufficient evidence*: Generally this evidence is provided by positive carcinogenicity studies in 2 or more species of animals or in 2 or more independent studies in one species but at different times and under different laboratory conditions. In exceptional cases, a single study in one species may provide sufficient evidence of carcinogenicity when the cancer occurs to an unusual degree with regard to incidence, site, type of tumour or age of onset.

(b) *Limited evidence*: Generally this evidence is provided by either positive carcinogenicity in a single experiment or unresolved questions regarding the adequacy of positive studies, or the agents or mixtures increase the incidence of only benign neoplasms or lesions of uncertain neoplastic potential (e.g., certain neoplasms may occur spontaneously in high incidence in certain strains of animals).

(c) *Inadequate evidence*: If studies cannot be interpreted as showing either the presence or absence of a carcinogenic effect, then the evidence for carcinogenicity is considered inadequate.

(d) *Evidence suggesting lack of carcinogenicity*: Generally this evidence is provided by adequate studies involving at least 2 species which show a lack of carcinogenicity. This evidence is limited to the species, tumour sites and levels of exposure studied.

Other similar classification schemes for carcinogens have been used. The US National Toxicology Program (NTP), for example, has somewhat different guidelines for classification of animal carcinogens [5], as does the US EPA.

Short-Term Bioassays for Genetic and Related Effects: The Mechanism of Cancer Induction

Evidence has been growing since the 1960s to support the theory that electrophilic chemicals react covalently with the nucleophilic centres in DNA and subsequently induce genetic changes (e.g., mutations). When such reactive electrophilic chemical mutagens react with DNA, this event may become the initiating event in a multistage process leading to cancer [6,7]. The mutational theory of cancer is supported by evidence that many electrophilic mutagens also induce cancer in animals [7]. The theory that the event which initiates cancer is caused by a genetic change in DNA, and the evidence supporting it, have become the basis for using short-term genetic bioassays to detect carcinogens.

There are, however, many aspects of the carcinogenic process which are unknown or only partly understood. There is growing evidence suggesting that different agents (e.g., chemicals or mixtures) may act at different stages in the carcinogenic process and by different mechanisms, including, in some cases, so-called non-genotoxic mechanisms [8-11]. This recognition has encouraged the scientific development of short-term bioassays for the detection of carcinogens which act at other stages in the cancer process. There are a number of short term bioassays which detect changes in cells that are not necessarily the result of genetic changes but that are thought to have specific relevance to the process of carcinogenesis. These bioassays include tests for tumour-promoting activity, cellular proliferation, intercellular communication and neoplastic cell transformation [6,12,13].

Short-term bioassays are often classified by the following phylogenetic groups: prokaryotes, fungi, plants, insects, mammalian cells (*in vitro*), mammalian cells (*in vivo*) and human (tissues/body fluids) [2,6,14]. Short-term bioassay data are evaluated and interpreted based on the biological endpoints detected which include the following: DNA damage, gene mutation, sister chromatid exchange, micronuclei, chromosomal aberrations, aneuploidy and cell transformation [14]. Some of these endpoints are more directly related to a genotoxic event (e.g., gene mutations and chromosomal aberrations), while others are less clearly genetic but may be related to changes in DNA (e.g., unscheduled DNA synthesis, formation of DNA adducts) or cellular changes related to both tumour initiation and progression or promotion (e.g., oncogenic cell transformation).

Predicting Cancer Risk Using Short-Term Bioassays

Many studies have evaluated the correlation between mutagenicity in short-term tests and carcinogenicity in animals. Studies of hundreds of chemicals in the 1970s demonstrated that bacterial mutagenicity assays detected over 90% of the animal carcinogens which had been identified up to that time [15-17]. Several changes occurred in the 1980s in rodent cancer bioassay protocols (e.g., testing up to the maximum tolerable dose, MTD) and the types of chemicals being tested [18]. The method of chemical selection was changed from selecting chemicals with electrophilic structures to high-volume industrial chemicals, because these chemicals may have greater potential for human exposure. A recent report on 73 such chemicals showed that short-term genetic bioassays only predicted about 60% of these animal carcinogens [19]. The conclusions of this study regarding the utility of short-term tests have raised many critical issues related to predicting cancer risk in humans based on experimental data in both animals and short-term bioassays [18,20-22]. These issues include: (1) concordance between carcinogenicity results in rats and mice and the concordance between these rodents and short-term genetic bioassays [20,22]; (2) influence of chemical class on the sensitivity and specificity of genetic bioassays [23]; and (3) genotoxic versus non-genotoxic carcinogens [24]. It is clear that animal carcinogens which are also mutagenic are more likely to be carcinogenic across species and target organs and are carcinogenic at much lower doses [25]. Bioassays that detect, by definition, genotoxic agents would not be expected to detect agents that may induce cancer by a mechanism which does not involve interaction with DNA; mutation induction or other genetic effects. The tumours induced by non-mutagenic chemicals tend to be limited to one species and organ site [18], although the data base for supporting this conclusion is not large. The human cancer risk of these non-genotoxic rodent carcinogens may be questionable, particularly if the agent induces tumours in only one species and only at the MTD [20,22]. Although the list of recognised human carcinogens [2] is much smaller than the list of animal carcinogens, most of these human carcinogenic agents are positive in short-term bioassays [4,21,26]. The chemicals which are rodent carcinogens across several species and organ sites (transspecies carcinogens) are generally also mutagenic in short-term bioassays [18,25].

Quantitative Assessment of Cancer Risk

The classification of carcinogens according to their mechanisms of action [8] could facilitate both the qualitative and quantitative assessment of cancer risk but, until recently, sufficient data on the mechanism of cancer induction by various agents was not known. Most international and national health and environmental agencies do not classify or regulate carcinogens according to their mechanisms of action. This may change in the future when a better understanding of carcinogenesis mechanisms is obtained. The organisations which conduct quantitative carcinogen risk assessments have only made some attempts to classify carcinogens by their mechanism of action (e.g., genotoxic versus non-genotoxic carcinogens) for the purpose of extrapolation modelling at low doses. For quantitative cancer risk assessment to be scientifically defensible in the future, an understanding of the mechanism of an agent's action in inducing cancer may be required [27,28].

Quantitative cancer risk assessments using linear or other non-threshold low-dose extrapolations are based on the assumptions that involve the genetic mechanism of cancer induction [8]. If it can be shown that a carcinogen acts by a non-genotoxic mechanism which results in a threshold dose below which no excess cancers would be observed, then linear non-threshold low-dose extrapolations may be inappropriate models. Quantitative cancer risk assessment as developed and applied by the US Environmental Protection Agency (EPA) in the 1980s [29] was based on a methodology developed by Crump [30] to estimate cancer risk from chronic animal experiments. This approach is referred to as the linearised multistage model and is widely used to establish upper bounds on suspected cancer risk. One of the important deficiencies of this model is that it is not derived from an underlying biological theory of carcinogenesis and does not take into account agent-induced stimulation of cell proliferation. A 2-stage model of carcinogenesis proposed by Armitage and Doll [31] was based on the biological evidence that stem cells are transformed into premalignant cells. They proposed that these premalignant cells divide at a constant rate, producing an exponential growth of preneoplastic clones. A preneoplastic cell is then transformed into a cancer cell, which may ultimately develop into a tumour. More recently, Moolgavkar and Knudson [32] have proposed a mathematical model which is based on the biological evidence linking mutation induction and tumour formation. This model assumes that the first critical event in a series of steps which can lead to cancer is the induction of a mutation in the DNA of a normal stem cell resulting in a preneoplastic cell. The second critical step is the transformation of a preneoplastic cell into a malignant cancer cell. Biologically motivated cancer risk models such as the 2-stage model have many advantages over purely mathematical approaches to risk assessment [33]. Importantly, the parameters in the model are interpretable in biological terms and may potentially be estimated from experimental cellular data, including mutation and cell-transformation data. Cell-proliferation and cellular-toxicity (death) data may also be incorporated into this model.

Individual Air Pollutant Chemicals

More than 2,800 different individual chemicals have been identified as atmospheric compounds [34]. These compounds represent almost every known chemical class. The number of chemicals identified in each class does not necessarily represent the distribution of chemicals by class in the air, since the chemicals which have been identified are highly dependent on our current chemical analytical detection methods. Graedel et al. [34] suggested that alcohols, carboxylic acids and nitrogen-containing organic compounds are underrepresented with respect to their actual occurrence in the ambient air. Table 1 shows the number of chemicals in each category that have been detected in atmospheres including ambient air, indoor air and air emission sources. Unfortunately, only about 10% of these chemicals have been evaluated in any bioassays. Table 1 shows the number of chemicals in each category for which either short-term bacterial genetic bioassay data or animal cancer data have been reported. Three categories (hydrocarbons, nitrogen-

Table 1. Occurrence and bioassay results for airborne chemicals

Category	Number of compounds identified	Number bioassayed	Positive compounds Type of Bioassay	
			Animal	STT*
Inorganics	260	30	4	5
Hydrocarbons	729	51	19	12
Ethers	44	3	0	1
Alcohols	233	28	0	1
Ketones	227	11	0	0
Aldehydes	108	6	1	4
Carboxylic acid derivatives	219	6	2	0
Carboxylic acids	174	5	0	0
Heterocyclic oxygen compounds	93	16	7	4
Nitrogen-containing organics	384	59	12	22
Sulphur-containing organics	99	4	1	1
Halogen-containing organics	216	71	21	16
Organometallic compounds	41	13	0	6
GRAND TOTALS	2827	303	67	72

* STT=short-term tests as described in the text   Adapted from Graedel et al. [34]

containing organics and halogenated organics) account for nearly 60% of the compounds that have been bioassayed. This table shows that the percentage of ketones, carboxylic acids and their derivatives which have been identified in the air is much greater than the percentage of those compounds with any bioassay data. Therefore, the contribution of these categories of chemicals to the potential airborne carcinogens cannot be estimated.

This computerised data base on the occurrence of atmospheric compounds has been merged with the largest evaluated bioassay data base. The bioassay data base was developed by the US Environmental Protection Agency Gene-Tox Program [14], with the assistance of many international experts who reviewed and evaluated the bioassay data. This entire bioassay data base contains bioassay results for 2,346 compounds, only 303 of which are overlapping with the 2,827 compounds that have been identified as air pollutants. As shown in Table 1, the 3 chemical categories which have the most bioassay data also have the highest number of positive bioassay results in both animal cancer tests and short-term bioassay tests. This data is very useful in summarising what is known and what is not known about the potential genotoxic and carcinogenic activity of compounds found in air pollution. Unfortunately, the distribution of both chemicals and positive bioassay results reflects the degree of attention paid by atmospheric chemists and toxicologists to specific classes of chemicals, rather than the degree of potential hazard of these classes of chemicals compared to those chemical classes which have not been investigated. This data base does not include the relative exposure concentrations of these chemicals; a critical factor in understanding the potential risk (See Chapter 3).

When the source of each atmospheric compound is included in the analysis of the occurrence of biologically active compounds, several conclusions become apparent [34]. Firstly, the sources which emit the highest number of bioassay-positive chemicals are sources involving combustion (e.g., tobacco smoke, automobile exhaust and coal combustion). Non-combustion sources including chemical manufacturing and pesticides are also significant, but in this analysis rank below the combustion sources. Vegetation appears on the list because of the low molecular weight aldehydes frequently emitted by plants (see Chapter 2).

Weight of Evidence for Human Cancer Risk of Individual Chemicals

The list of chemicals identified in air has been combined with the weight of evidence for carcinogenic risks to humans for those chemicals by the IARC evaluation [35] as shown in Table 2. Of those chemicals with sufficient evidence for human carcinogenicity, benzene is the one chemical with the highest and best characterised human exposure (see Chapter 3). Of those chemicals with limited evidence for human carcinogenicity but sufficient evidence for animal carcinogenicity (Group 2A), formaldehyde has the highest and best characterised human exposure. Of the other chemicals in the Group 2A and 2B category (sufficient evidence for animal carcinogenicity) identified in air with human exposure assessment data, the following have been identified as potentially important contributors to human cancer risk: 1,3-butadiene, chloroform, ethylene dibromide and carbon tetrachloride [35,36].

There are many uncertainties in evaluating the weight of evidence for human cancer risk of the chemicals found in air pollution. One of the most important of these is that other chemicals, either not yet identified in air or not studied in animal cancer or short-term bioassays, may eventually be shown to be more significant air pollutants in the future. There is recent evidence from studies of complex mixtures of urban air particles and gases that the major contributors to the genotoxic activity of urban air are mutagens which have not yet been identified and may be produced upon atmospheric transformation of organics emitted by many sources [37,38]. New bioassay-directed chemical identification techniques have identified polar organic species (e.g., hydroxylated and nitrated aromatic hydrocarbons) in urban air [37] (see Chapter 2).

Table 2. Summary of the weight of evidence for human cancer risk of individual airborne chemicals

CHEMICAL	Evidence for Carcinogenicity			
	HUMAN [a]	ANIMAL [a]	STT [b]	OVERALL [c] EVALUATION
ARSENIC and ARSENIC COMPOUNDS	S	S	+	1
BENZENE	S	S	+	1
BIS(CHLOROMETHYL)ETHER	S	S	+	1
CHLOROMETHYL METHYL ETHER	S	S	+	1
CHROMIUM (VI) COMPOUNDS	S	S	+	1
NICKEL and NICKEL COMPOUNDS	S	S	+	1
VINYL CHLORIDE	S	S	+	1
ACRYLONITRILE	L	S	+	2A
BERYLLIUM (OXIDE) CPDS	L	S	+	2A
Cd (II) OXIDE	L	S	(+)	2A
EPOXYETHANE	L	S	+	2A
FORMALDEHYDE	L	S	+	2A
DIMETHYL SULFATE	I	S	+	2A
DIBROMOETHYLENE	I	S	+	2A
EPOXYPROPANE, 1,2-	I	S	+	2A
EPICHLOROHYDRIN	I	S	+	2A
BENZO (A) PYRENE	ND	S	+	2A
DIBENZ (A,H) ANTHRACENE	ND	S	+	2A
N-NITROSODIMETHYLAMINE	ND	S	+	2A
ACETALDEHYDE	I	S	+	2B
BUTADIENE, 1,3-	I	S	+	2B
CARBON TETRACHLORIDE	I	S	(+)	2B
CHLOROFORM	I	S	(-)	2B
DICHLOROPROPANE, 1,3-	I	S	+	2B
DIOXANE, 1,4-	I	S	(-)	2B
HYDRAZINE	I	S	+	2B
LEAD (INORGANIC)	I	S	(-)	2B
STYRENE	I	L	+	2B
VINYLIDENE CHLORIDE	I	L	+	3
BENZO (J) FLUORANTHENE	ND	S	(+)	2B
DIBENZO (A,E) PYRENE	ND	S	(+)	2B
DIBENZO (A,L) PYRENE	ND	S	ND	2B
DIBENZO (C,G) CARBAZOLE	ND	S	ND	2B
DIBENZ (A,H) ACRIDINE	ND	S	(+)	2B
DIBENZ (A,J) ACRIDINE	ND	S	+	2B
DICHLOROETHANE, 1,2-	ND	S	+-	2B
DIMETHYLHYDRAZINE	ND	S	+	2B
DINITROPYRENE, 1,6-	ND	S	+	2B
DINITROPYRENE, 1,8-	ND	S	+	2B
INDENO (1,2,3-CD) PYRENE	ND	S	(+)	2B

Table 2. (continued)

| CHEMICAL | Evidence for Carcinogenicity | | | |
	HUMAN [a]	ANIMAL [a]	STT [b]	OVERALL [c] EVALUATION
NITROCHRYSENE, 6-	ND	S	+	2B
NITROFLUORENE, 2-	ND	S	+	2B
NITROPROPANE, 2-	ND	S	+	2B
NITROPYRENE, 1-	ND	S	+	2B
NITROPYRENE, 4-	ND	S	+	2B
N-NITROSODIETHANOLAMINE	ND	S	+	2B
N-NITROSOMORPHOLINE	ND	S	+	2B

a   Degree of Evidence as evaluated by IARC (1987-1989) in the following categories:

S = Sufficient evidence of carcinogenicity as evaluated by IARC

L = Limited evidence of carcinogenicity as evaluated by IARC

I = Inadequate evidence of carcinogenicity as evaluated by IARC

ND = No adequate data

b   STT = Short term tests for genotoxicity, mutagenicity or cell transformation. This evidence has been summarised into + to indicate positive results, - to indicate negative results or () to indicate an inconclusive evaluation with either both + and - studies reported or an insufficient number of adequate STT to evaluate.

c   Overall Evaluation category by Groups as evaluated by IARC (1987-1989):

Group 1 = carcinogenic to humans

Group 2A = probably carcinogenic to humans

Group 2B = possily carcinogenic to humans

Group 3 = not classifiable as to carcinogenicity to humans

Group 4 = probably NOT carcinogenic to humans (none listed)

Quantitative Estimates of the Contribution of Individual Chemicals to Human Cancer Risk

Quantitation of cancer risk from individual chemicals in air has many uncertainties associated with both the exposure assessment and cancer potency assessment which are combined to produce an estimate of excess cancer cases. In spite of these large uncertainties, this procedure is being widely used in the US to rank the importance of chemicals and sources associated with air pollution [36]. The total annual number of cancer cases for the US estimated to be derived from outdoor air is approximately 2,000 cases per year, which is similar in magnitude to the estimated number of cancer cases from passive smoking and much less than the number of cancer deaths in the US attributed to cigarette smoking. This analysis has many uncertainties and does not include in the analysis all possible sources or all chemicals that have been identified in the air, as discussed above. Figure 1 illustrates the relative contribution of a number of individual chemicals and several mixtures to the total estimated US cancer cases per year from outdoor air pollutants using this method [36]. The most dramatic observation from this analysis is the estimated importance of products of incomplete combustion (PIC), which is a very complex mixture of gases and particles. The other major contributing chemicals in this analysis include several which are either evaluated by IARC as having sufficient evidence (Group 1) to be carcinogenic to humans or are probably (2A) or possibly (2B) carcinogenic to humans,

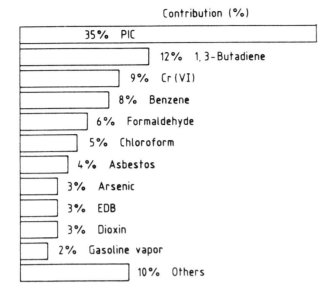

Fig. 1. Relative contribution of airborne chemicals to the estimated carcinogenic load due to outdoor air pollution in the US [36]

including: 1,3-butadiene, benzene, formaldehyde, chloroform, asbestos, ethylene dibromide and carbon tetrachloride. Of the remaining chemicals which this analysis estimates may be important, there are several where the weight of evidence for human cancer risk is lacking, principally through a lack of animal bioassay data. Those chemicals include several inorganic compounds: hexavalent chromium and arsenic.

Mixtures of Air Pollutants

The first recognised chemical carcinogens were the coal tars and soots from chimneys, which were found to induce not only scrotal cancer in humans but tumours in animals [39]. It is now known that combustion, pyrolysis and other types of thermal treatment of organic matter, result in the formation of polycyclic aromatic compounds (PACs) such as the polycyclic aromatic hydrocarbon (PAH), benzo(a)pyrene. Many individual PACs are carcinogenic in animals (see Table 2) and genotoxic in short-term tests [40]. Humans, however, are not generally exposed to individual PACs, but to complex mixtures containing these compounds. These and other mixtures of air pollutants will be discussed as (a) mixtures from sources emitted into the air and (b) mixtures of air pollution as they occur in urban, industrial, rural and indoor air.

Source Mixtures

Many of the mixtures found in air which are listed in Table 3 as having an overall evaluation as carcinogenic to humans (Category 1), had sufficient evidence for excess cancer risk in humans exposed through occupational exposures (e.g., coke production, iron and steel founding). The industrial mixtures listed in Table 3 may not all have significant emissions to the outdoor air (e.g., boot and shoe manufacturing and repair). Several of these industrial sources are either not widely found or are not currently practised throughout the world (e.g., shale oils and coal gasification). Other industrial source emissions can be significant sources of air pollution in industrial areas where they are present (e.g., coke production, iron and steel founding, aluminum production, lumber and paper industries). Two of these Category 1 carcinogens are primarily indoor air pollutants: asbestos and tobacco smoke.

The most widely distributed outdoor air pollutant is soot. Soot is a mixture of sub-micron carbonacous particles which contain a relatively high percentage of condensed organic matter (tar). Although the first soot to be recognised as a human carcinogen was the soot from coal combustion [41], there is increasing evidence that soots from the combustion of other fuels (e.g., petroleum, wood) are similar in their composition, genetic activity and induction of tumours in animals [42,43]. A recent IARC evaluation of diesel and petrol engine exhausts relied heavily on the animal evidence of carcinogenicity to evaluate these mixtures as probably and possibly carcinogenic to humans [44] (see Table 3). Vehicular emissions from automobiles, buses, trucks and other mobile sources are ubiquitous air pollutants in urban areas. Quantitative estimates of the possible contribution to human cancer risk in the United States suggest approximately half of the estimated cancer risk from outdoor air pollution may result from exposure to motor vehicle

Table 3. Summary of the weight of evidence for human cancer risk of airborne pollutant mixtures

| MIXTURES | Evidence for Carcinogenicity | | | |
	HUMAN [a]	ANIMAL [a]	STT [b]	OVERALL [c] EVALUATION
ASBESTOS	S	S	(+)	1
COAL-TAR PITCHES	S	S	+	1
COAL-TARS	S	S	+	1
SHALE OILS	S	S	+	1
TOBACCO SMOKE	S	S	+	1
RUBBER INDUSTRY	S	I	+	1
SOOTS	S	I	+	1
FURNITURE and CABINET MAKING	S	I	ND	1
ALUMINUM PRODUCTION	S		+	1
BOOT and SHOE MANUFACTURE and REPAIR	S		ND	1
COAL GASIFICATION	S		+	1
COKE PRODUCTION	S		+	1
IRON and STEEL FOUNDING	S		+	1
DIESEL				
WHOLE DIESEL ENGINE EXHAUST	L	S	+	2A
GAS-PHASE DIESEL ENGINE EXHAUST (PARTICLES REMOVED)		I	(+)	
EXTRACTS OF PARTICLES		S	+	
PETROL				
WHOLE PETROL ENGINE EXHAUST	I	I	+	2B
CONDENSATES/EXTRACTS OF PETROL ENGINE EXHAUST		S	+	
ENGINE EXHAUSTS (UNSPECIFIED)	L		+	
LUMBER & SAWMILL INDUSTRIES (INCLUDING LOGGING)	I		ND	3
PULP and PAPER MANUFACTURING	I		+	3

a   Degree of Evidence as evaluatuated by IARC (1987-1989) in the following categories:

S = Sufficient evidence of carcinogenicity as evaluated by IARC ·

L = Limited evidence of carcinogenicity as evaluated by IARC

I = Inadequate evidence of carcinogenicity as evaluated by IARC

ND = No adequate data

b   STT = Short term tests for genotoxicity, mutagenicity or cell transformation. This evidence has been summarised into + to indicate positive results, - to indicate negative results or () to indicate an inconclusive evaluation with either both + and - studies reported or an insufficient number of adequate STT to evaluate.

c   Overall Evaluation category by Groups as evaluated by IARC (1987-1989):

Group 1 = carcinogenic to humans

Group 2A = probably carcinogenic to humans

Group 2B = possibly carcinogenic to humans

Group 3 = not classifiable as to carcinogenicity to humans

Group 4 = probably NOT carcinogenic to humans (none listed)

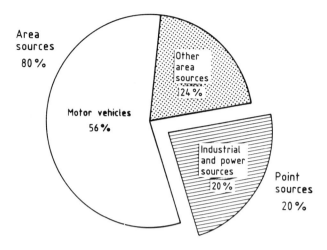

Fig. 2. Relative contribution of source categories to the estimated cancer cases due to outdoor air pollution sources in the US [36]

emissions and another one-fourth of the risk from other area sources [36], as illustrated in Figure 2.

Urban Air Mixtures

Particulate matter collected from the ambient air contains condensed organic matter similar to that described above for soot. A number of studies have shown that this organic extractable matter from air particles is carcinogenic in animals [45-47] and mutagenic in short-term bioassays [37,48-50]. Short-term mutagenicity bioassays have been used in ambient air monitoring studies and chemical characterisation studies in order to identify the major sources and compounds which contribute to the mutagenic activity of air particulate extracts [37,51]. Small area combustion sources, which include vehicles and home heating sources, have been shown to account for most of the mutagenic activity associated with air particulate matter in many urban areas [52], whereas in highly industrialised areas there is evidence of a significant contribution by coke ovens and other sources known to emit significant quantities of mutagenic polycyclic organic matter [53].

Gaseous mixtures of air pollutants studied in short-term mutagenesis bioassays in plants and bacteria are mutagenic, particularly after atmospheric transformations [54-56]. These studies suggest that highly reactive nitrogen-containing gases, such as peroxyacetyl nitrate (PAN), formed from ozone and nitrogen oxides reacting with simple non-mutagenic hydrocarbons, may produce genotoxic gases present in the urban air. Atmospheric transformations by ozone and nitrogen oxides have also been shown to increase the mutagenic activity of particulate matter and alter the nature of the mutagens to form more polar mutagens, including nitroarenes [57].

Summary

Experimental evidence in animal studies and short-term bioassays provides much of the evidence that certain air pollutants are carcinogenic. Of the nearly 3,000 chemicals identified, so far, as air pollutants, only 10% have been studied in experimental bioassays. Many of the chemicals or mixtures which are carcinogenic to humans also induce tumours in animals and are genotoxic in short-term bioassays. There are many more air pollutants which have been shown to be carcinogenic in animals for which no adequate human data are available. In some cases, human data for the individual chemicals may never be obtained, since humans are only exposed to mixtures of these chemicals (e.g., PAH). In the absence of such human data, it is advisable to regard these air pollutants as presenting a carcinogenic risk to humans. There are many more air pollutants which have only been evaluated in short-term bioassays. The prediction of cancer risk based only on positive short-term tests is less certain, however, in the absence of other data, it would be advisable to avoid excessive and prolonged exposure to such agents.

Of all the air pollutants studied in humans and experimental systems, the greatest human exposure and risk appears to be associated with mixtures of polycyclic aromatic compounds, particularly those derived from incomplete combustion. The sources of greatest concern in urban areas are usually the area sources such as motor vehicles and residential heating, due to the high human exposure resulting from their proximity to population centres. In certain industrial areas, however, coke ovens, aluminum smelters, iron and steel foundries, chemical plants, power plants and other industrial sources have been shown to emit significant quantities of carcinogenic agents into the air.

Acknowledgement

The author aknowledges the assistance of Katherine Williams in the preparation of Tables 2 and 3. The research described in this paper has been reviewed by the Health Effects Research Laboratory, U.S. Environmental Protection Agency and approved for publication. Approval does not signify that the contents necessarily reflect the views and policies of the Agency.

REFERENCES

1   Higginson J, Jensen OM: Epidemiological review of lung cancer in man. In: Mohr U, Schmahl D, Tomatis L (eds) Air Pollution and Cancer in Man. IARC Scientific Publications No. 16. International Agency for Research on Cancer, Lyon 1977 pp 169-189

2   IARC: IARC Monographs on the Evaluation of Carcinogenic Risks to Humans, Suppl 7. Overall Evaluations of Carcinogenicity: An Updating of IARC Monographs Volumes 1- 42. International Agency for Research on Cancer, Lyon 1987 pp 17-34

3   Wilbourn J, Haroun L, Heseltine E, Kaldor J, Partensky C, Vainio H: Response of experimental animals to human carcinogens: An analysis based upon the IARC Monographs Programme. Carcinogenesis 1986 (7):1853-1863

4   Tomatis L, Aitio, A, Wilbourn, J and Shuker L: Human carcinogens so far identified. Jpn J Cancer Res 1989 (80):795-807

5   Huff JE, McConnell EE, Haseman, JK, Boorman, GA, Eustis SL, Schwartz BA, Rao GN, Jameson CK, Hart LG, and Rall DP: Carcinogenesis studies: results of 398 experiments on 104 chemicals from the US National Toxicology Program. Ann NY Acad Sci 1988 (534):1-30

6   Montesano R, Bartch H, Vainio H, Wilbourn J, Yamasaki H (Eds) Long-Term and Short-Term Assays for Carcinogenesis - A Critical Appraisal, IARC Scientific Publications No. 83. International Agency for Research on Cancer, Lyon 1986

7   Miller EC, Miller JA: The mutagenicity of chemical carcinogens: Correlations, problems, and interpretations. In Hollaender A (ed) Chemical Mutagens: Principles and Methods for Their Detection, Vol. 1. Plenum Press, New York 1971 pp 83-94

8   IARC: Approaches to Classifying Chemical Carcinogens According to Mechanism of Action. IARC Internal Technical Report 1983 No. 83/001

9   Yamasaki H: Multistage carcinogenesis: implications for risk estimation. Cancer Metastasis Rev 1988 (7):5-18

10 Farber E: Cellular biochemistry of the stepwise development of cancer with chemicals: GHA Clowes Memorial Lecture. Cancer Res 1984 (44):5463

11 Farber E: Possible etiologic mechanisms in chemical carcinogenesis. Environ Health Perspect 1987 (75):65

12 Butterworth BE and Slaga TU: A perspective on cell proliferation in rodent carcinogenicity studies: relevance to human beings. In: Chemically Induced Cell Proliferation: Implications for Risk Assessment. Wiley/Liss, New York 1989 (in press)

13 Trosko JE and Chang CC: Non-genotoxic mechanisms in carcinogenesis: role of inhibited intercellular communication. In: Hart RW and Hoerger FD (eds) Carcinogen Risk Assessment, Banbury Report 31. Cold Spring Harbor Laboratory, Cold Spring Harbor, New York 1988 pp139-174

14 Waters, MD, Auletta, A: The GENE-TOX program: genetic activity evaluation. J Chem Inf Comput Sci 1981(21):35-38

15 McCann J, Choi E, Yamasaki E and Ames BN: Detection of carcinogens as mutagens in the Salmonella/microsome test: Assay of 300 chemicals. Proc Natl Acad Sci USA 1975 (72):5135-5139

16 Bartsch H: Predictive value of mutagenicity tests in chemical carcinogenesis. Mutat Res 1976 (38):177-190

17 Sugimura TS, Sato M, Nagao T, Yahagi T, Matsushima Y, Seino M, Takeuch and Kawachi T: Overlapping of carcinogens and mutagens. In: Magee PN, Takayama S, Sugimura T and Matsushima T (eds) Fundamentals of Cancer Prevention. University Park Press, Baltimore MD 1976 pp191-213

18 Ashby J and Tennant RW: Chemical structure, salmonella mutagenicity and extent of carcinogenicity as indicators of genotoxic carcinogenesis among 222 chemicals tested in rodents of the U.S. NCI/NTP Mutat Res 1988 (204):17-115

19 Tennant RW, Margolin BH, Shelby MD, Zeiger E, Haseman JK, Spalding, J, Caspary W, Resnick M, Stasiewicz S, Anderson B, Minor R: Prediction of chemical carcinogenicity in rodents from in vitro genetic toxicity assays. Science 1987 (236):933-941

20 Brockman HE and DeMarini DM: Utility of short-term tests for genetic toxicity in the aftermath of the NTP's analysis of 73 chemicals. Environ Mol Mutagen 1988 (11):421-435

21 Bartch H and Malaveille C: Prevalence of genotoxic chemicals among animal and human carcinogens evaluated in the IARC Monograph Series. Cell Biol Toxicol 1989 (5):115-127

22 Lave LB, Ennever FK, Rosenkranz HS and Omenn GS: Information value of the rodent bioassay. Nature 1988 (336):431-433

23 Claxton LD, Stead AG and Walsh D: An analysis by chemical class of Salmonella mutagenicity tests as predictors of animal carcinogenicity. Mutat Res 1988 (205):197-225

24 Ashby J: The separate identities of genotoxic and non-genotoxic carcinogens. Mutagenesis 1988 (3):365-366

25 Gold LS, Slone TH, Backman GM, Eisenberg S, DaCosta M, Wong M, Manley, NB, Rohrbach L, and Ames BN: Third chronological supplement to the carcinogenic potency database: Standardized results of animal bioassays published through December 1986 and by the National Toxicology Program through June 1987. Environ Health Perspect 1989 (84)

26 Garrett, NE, Stack, HF, Gross, MR, Waters, MD: An analysis of the spectra of genetic activity produced by known or suspected human carcinogens. Mutat Res 1984 (134):89-111

27 Ames BM, Magaw R and Gold LS: Ranking possible carcinogenic hazards. Science 1987 (236):271

28 Ames BN, Magaw R and Gold LS: Response to letter: Risk assessment. Science 1987 (237):235

29 Anderson EL and the Cancer Assessment Group of the US Environmental Protection Agency: Quantitative approaches in use to assess cancer risk. Risk Anal 1983 (3):277-295

30 Crump KS: An improved procedure for low-dose carcinogenic risk assessment from animal data. J Environ Pathol Toxicol 1981 (5):675-684

31 Armitage P and Doll R: A two-stage theory of carcinogenesis in relation to the age distribution of human cancer. Br J Cancer 1957 (11):161-169

32 Moolgavkar SH and Knudson AG: Mutation and cancer: A model for human carcinogenesis. JNCI 1981 (66):1037-1052

33 Thorslund TW, Brown CC and Charnley G: Biologically motivated cancer risk models. Risk Anal 1987 (7):109-119

34 Graedel, TE, Hawkins, DT, Claxton, LD: Atmospheric Chemical Compounds: Sources, Occurrence, and Bioassay. Academic Press Inc, Orlando FL 1986 p 732

35 IARC: IARC Monographs on the Evaluation of Carcinogenic Risks to Humans, Volumes 1-46. International Agency for Research on Cancer, Lyon

36 US Environmental Protection Agency: Cancer Risk from Outdoor Exposure to Air Toxics. Office of Air Quality Planning and Standards, Research Triangle Park, NC 27711. EPA-450/2-89

37 Lewtas J: Genotoxicity of complex mixtures: strategies for the identification and comparative assessment of airborne mutagens and carcinogens from combustion sources. Fundam Appl Toxicol 1988 (10):571-589

38 Claxton, LD: Assessment of bacterial bioassay methods for volatile and semivolatile compounds and mixtures. Environ Int 1985 (11):375-382

39 Searle CE (ed) Chemical Carcinogens. ACS Monograph No 173. American Chemical Society, Washington DC 1976

40 IARC: IARC Monographs on the Evaluation of Carcinogenic Risks to Humans, Polynuclear Aromatic Compounds. Part 1, Chemical, Environmental and Experimental Data. Vol 32. International Agency for Research on Cancer, Lyon 1983

41 IARC: IARC Monographs on the Evaluation of Carcinogenic Risks to Humans, Polynuclear Aromatic Compounds. Part 4, Bitumens, Coal-tar and Derived Products, Shale Oils and Soots. Vol 35. International Agency for Research on Cancer, Lyon 1985

42 Hoffman, D, Wynder, EL: Environmental respiratory carcinogenesis. In: Searle CE (ed) Chemical Carcinogens. ACS Monograph 173. American Chemical Society, Washington DC 1976 (7): 324-365

43 Lewtas J: Combustion emissions: Characterization and comparison of their mutagenic and carcinogenic activity. In: HF Stich (ed) Carcinogens and Mutagens in the Environment. Vol V, The Workplace. CRC Press, Boca Raton F, 1985 pp 59-74

44 IARC: IARC Monographs on the Evaluation of Carcinogenic Risks to Humans. Diesel and Gasoline Engine Exhausts and Some Nitroarenes. Vol 46. International Agency for Research on Cancer, Lyon 1989

45 Leiter J, Shimkin MB, Shear MJ: Production of subcutaneous sarcomas in mice with tars extracted from atmospheric dusts. J Natl Cancer Inst 1942 (3):155-165

46 Kotin P, Falk HL, Mader P, Thomas M: Aromatic hydrocarbons. 1. Presence in the Los Angeles atmosphere and the carcinogenicity of atmospheric extracts. Arch Indust Hyg 1954 (9):153-163

47 Hueper WC, Kotin P, Tabor EC, Payne W, Falk HL, Sawiciki E: Carcinogenic bioassays on air pollutants. Arch Pathol 1962 (74):89-116

48 Alfheim I, Lofroth G, Moller M: Bioassay of extracts of ambient particulate matter. Environ Health Persp 1983 (47):227-238

49 Matsushita H, Goto S, Takagi Y: Human exposure to airborne mutagens indoors and outdoors using mutagenesis and chemical analysis methods. In: Waters M, Lewtas J, Nesnow S, Moore M, Daniel FB (eds) Short-Term Bioassays in the Analysis of Complex Environmental Mixtures VI. Plenum Press, New York 1990 (in press)

50 Barale R, Migliore L, Cellini B, Francioni L, Giogelli F, Barai I, Loprieno N: Genetic toxicology of airborne particulate matter using cytogenetic assays and microbial mutagenicity assays. In: Waters M, Lewtas J, Nesnow S, Moore M, Daniel FB (eds) Short-Term Bioassays in the Analysis of Complex Environmental Mixtures VI. Plenum Press, New York 1990 (in press)

51 Schuetzle D, Lewtas J: Bioassay-directed chemical analysis in environmental research. Anal Chem 1986 (58):1060A-1075A

52 Lewis CW, Baumgardner RE, Claxton LD, Lewtas J, Stevens RK: The contribution of woodsmoke and motor vehicle emissions to ambient aerosol mutagenicity. Environ Sci Technol 1988 (22):968-971

53 Tokiwa H, Morita K, Takeyoshi H, Takahashi K, Ohnishi Y: Detection of mutagenic activity in particulate air pollutants. 1977 Mutat Res (48):237-248

54 Tice RR, Costa DL, Schaich KM: Genotoxic Effects of Airborne Agents Vol 25, Environmental Science Research. Plenum Press, New York 1980

55 Claxton LD, Kleindienst TE, Perry E and Cupitt LT: Assessment of the mutagenicity of organic air pollutants before and after atmospheric transformation. In: Waters M, Lewtas J, Nesnow S, Moore M, Daniel FB (eds) Short-Term Bioassays in the Analysis of Complex Environmental Mixtures VI. Plenum Press, New York 1990 (in press)

56 Kleindienst TE, Shepson PB, Edney EO, Claxton LD, Cupitt LT: Wood smoke: measurement of the mutagenic activities of its gas-and particulate-phase photooxidation products. Environ Sci Technol 1986 (20): 493-501

57 Kamens RM, Rives GD, Perry JM, Bell DA, Paylor RF, Goodman RG, Claxton LD: Mutagenic changes in dilute wood smoke as it ages and reacts with ozone and nitrogen dioxide: An outdoor chamber study. Environ Sci Technol 1984 (7):523-530

Epidemiological Evidence on Air Pollution and Cancer

Göran Pershagen [1] and Lorenzo Simonato [2]

1 Institute of Environmental Medicine, Karolinska Institute, Box 60209, 104 01 Stockholm, Sweden
2 Centre of Environmental Carcinogenesis, University of Padova, via Facciolati 71, 35100 Padova, Italy

Introduction

Ambient air pollution may give rise to several types of effects on health. These range from reactions of annoyance and acute irritation of eyes and airways, to chronic inflammatory diseases, cancer and death [1]. Only malignant diseases will be discussed in this chapter, although it is realised that cancer may not represent the most important type of effect from a public health point of view.

The effects of air pollution on health may be due to direct exposure to pollutants or occur via indirect pathways. One example of indirect routes includes health effects related to increased exposure to heavy metals, which are more easily mobilised as a result of acidification of soil and water. In some areas, air pollution is a major contributor to acidification. Another example is skin cancer induced by ultraviolet radiation, which may increase due to the depletion of the ozone layer for which some air pollutants may be of importance. Such indirect effects of air pollution will not be considered here.

This chapter focusses on cancer risks related to exposure to ambient air pollution. Such exposure may take place both outdoors and indoors. The main emphasis is on air pollution in urban and industrialised areas. Exposure to primary sources indoors, e.g., radon or environmental tobacco smoke, and various occupational exposures will only be treated as possible confounders and/or effect modifiers. Lung cancer risks have received the greatest attention and these data are evaluated most thoroughly.

Lung Cancer

Descriptive Studies

The relationship between lung cancer and air pollution has been investigated in different countries through different methodological approaches. A large number of descriptive studies is available from the literature, which contributes an important body of knowledge to this issue. Descriptive studies are, however, limited because of 3 main problems:

- The exposure either at population or individual level is very difficult to assess. Air pollution is, in fact, a particularly complex mixture of chemicals and other substances which are rapidly modified by different atmospheric conditions and which, in addition, can interact with each other (see Chapter 2).
- Descriptive and correlation studies examine the effects at group level (e.g., population resident in a town) and it is not possible to assess whether individuals affected by the disease investigated are those actually exposed or "more exposed".
- Particularly for lung cancer, there are important confounding factors like tobacco smoke and occupational exposure which may contribute to an apparent association between air pollution and lung cancer risk. Information on confounding factors is generally not available in descriptive studies.

These limitations should induce caution when interpreting descriptive studies, due to the possibility of both false-positive and false-negative results. The former situation is generally due to the lack of control of confounding factors, while the latter is related to the low sensitivity of the studies due to the imprecision of the information on exposure at the individual level.

An important section of the epidemiological evidence supporting the hypothesis of a carcinogenic risk related to exposure to air pollutants comes from descriptive studies investigating urban/rural differences of lung cancer rates. The major limitation to a definite evaluation of these studies probably resides in the overwhelming effect of tobacco smoke and, to a lesser extent, occupational exposure to lung carcinogens. Tobacco smoke may increase the incidence of lung tumours up to 20 or 30 times in heavy smokers as compared to non-smokers. The increase is proportional to the average number of cigarettes smoked and is inversely related to the age of starting the habit. If we consider that the differences in lung cancer rates between urban and rural areas are, in general, around 100%, while even small variations in the amount smoked or in the age at which smoking was started can result in 3- to 5-fold increases, we can estimate, at least in part, the urban-rural gradient as effected by historical differences in the diffusion of smoking habits. There is evidence that smoking habits in many European countries have increased more rapidly in urban than in rural populations. Still in the 1970s, in England, the average cigarette consumption per capita in urban areas was 12 and 6 cigarettes/day in males and females, respectively, as compared to 5 and 3 in rural areas [2].

Several studies suggested an association between lung cancer and air pollution from the observation of an urban/rural gradient in lung cancer risk. In most of the countries from which mortality or incidence data for lung cancer were available in the 1950s and 1960s, the rates were 2 to 3 times higher in urban areas than in rural areas [3-7]. Stocks [3,8] observed that the mortality rate was higher in large towns than in small ones and that there was a correlation with the density of the population. The existence of an "urban factor" was subsequently supported by the results of numerous other descriptive studies [9,10]. Goldsmith [11] analysed U.S. mortality data during 1950-1960 in males, comparing urban and rural counties for a number of cancer sites. The results indicate a 2-fold ra-

tio for lung cancer between urban and rural populations. Trichopoulos et al. [12] conducted an epidemiological study comparing the mortality from lung cancer in Athens during the period 1961-1980 with the pattern of mortality from the same tumour in other Greek towns that are known to be much less affected by air pollution. The results did not indicate any effect of air pollution, either independent from or interactive with smoking, on the population resident in Athens.

The urban/rural gradient has been reduced progressively in the last 20 years. However, the gradient still exists and is evident in most of the countries from which data are available. Some examples of lung cancer rates from rural and urban areas are reported in Table 1. The data appear somewhat conflicting, judging from similar patterns in areas with a different history of air pollution, such as the U.K. and Norway. Furthermore, the relative urban excess in females does not appear fully consistent across countries.

Additional evidence provided by descriptive epidemiological studies which might be of help in estimating the upper limit of the carcinogenic effect of air pollution on lung cancer comes from a comparison of the rates of this tumour in males and females. Until the 1960s and 1970s, the lung cancer rates were 5 to 15 times higher in males than in females. Recent statistics show that lung cancer rates tend to level off among males while they are rapidly increasing among females. The phenomenon is somewhat conflicting with the pattern of air pollution exposures which have decreased, at least in England and the U.S., since the end of the 1950s. Thus, these two different trends of lung cancer rates in males and females appear unrelated to changes in exposure to air pollutants and are generally interpreted as the result of the different changes in smoking habits in the two sexes.

An attempt has been made to assess trends of lung cancer mortality in relation to reduction in air pollution, particularly in England and Wales in the 1920s and subsequently after the Clear Air Act of 1956. The major studies on this issue, e.g., those by the Royal College of Physicians [14] and by Lawther and Waller [15], suggest a beneficial effect on the lung cancer risk from the improved control of air pollution. The data do not take into ac-

Table 1. Age-standardised rates per 100,000 population for mortality from carcinoma of the bronchus and trachea in urban and rural areas *

Registry	Males			Females		
	Urban	Rural	Ratio	Urban	Rural	Ratio
Japan, Miyagi	30.9	28.4	1.1	9.2	8.1	1.1
Czechoslovakia, Slovakia	68.2	70.5	1.0	9.4	6.5	1.4
FRG, Saarland	77.7	63.0	1.2	7.7	6.0	1.3
France, Calvados	46.1	39.6	1.2	3.4	2.9	1.2
France, Doubs	56.9	40.1	1.4	3.3	2.0	1.7
Hungary, Szabolcs	61.8	50.9	1.2	10.3	6.2	1.7
Norway	39.4	24.5	1.6	9.6	5.2	1.9
Romania, Cluj County	35.2	35.3	1.0	6.7	4.7	1.4
Switzerland, Vaud	63.8	56.6	1.1	8.7	5.6	1.6
U.K., England and Wales	74.8	56.2	1.3	19.7	15.1	1.3
Australia, New South Wales	55.5	46.8	1.2	12.2	8.3	1.5

*   From IARC [13]

count, however, changes in cigarette usage and in tar content occurring during the same period.

Epidemiological investigations have been performed on migrants from areas characterised by high levels of air pollution to other areas or countries. Most of these studies were carried out in the 1950s and 1960s within countries of the British Commonwealth, i.e., British citizens migrating to Australia, New Zealand or South Africa. The results tend to show that British citizens migrating to countries with lower levels of air pollution had higher lung cancer rates than the local white population [16-18]. Some of these studies collected information on smoking habits of lung cancer cases and controls born in England and Wales as well as in the countries of emigration, showing that no major differeces in smoking habits were present between immigrants from the U.K. and the local white population. The authors of these studies concluded that the higher mortality due to lung cancer should be ascribed to exposure to air pollutants before emigration. The evidence was strengthened by the observation that the mortality excess was larger among individuals leaving the country after the age of 30 compared with those emigrating at a younger age. The studies are consistent in

indicating a lung cancer excess of around 40%.

In some respects, the most eligible population for studying the potential carcinogenic effects of air pollution are non-smokers, although recent epidemiological evidence strongly suggests a lung cancer risk from environmental tobacco smoke. The need to adjust also for this potential confounder further complicates the study design of the epidemiological research on the effects of air pollution. No relevant difference in lung cancer rates was found by Doll [19] between non-smokers resident in Greater London, other urban areas and rural districts. Mortality data for England and Wales have been subsequently analysed by Doll [20], who suggested a possible effect on lung cancer risk in relation to exposure to carcinogens in urban areas. The effect is believed to be small but an interactive effect with smoking and occupational exposure cannot be excluded.

Based on the State of Utah Cancer Registry, Lyon et al. [21] identified male and female lung cancer cases diagnosed from 1967 to 1975 among Mormons (who do not smoke or drink alcohol) and non-Mormons. Lung cancer incidence rate ratios in urban vs rural areas were estimated at 1.8 and 1.2 for men and women among non-Mormons. For

Mormons the corresponding rate ratios were 0.9 and 1.0.

Overall descriptive and correlation studies investigating the possible role of air pollution on the aetiology of lung cancer do not provide consistent results and do not permit firm conclusions. Although most of the studies show some association between lung cancer and air pollution, the lack of control for confounding factors, together with the highly imprecise definition of exposure, makes it difficult to interpret the data in quantitative terms.

Studies on Populations in Industrial Areas

Populations living in areas close to industries suspected of contributing heavily to air pollution have been studied to ascertain any increased risk of lung cancer which could be related to air pollution. Most of these studies are of ecological character and often limited by a lack of information on smoking habits and occupational exposures. With few exceptions, these studies did not have access to detailed information on exposure patterns (particularly historical) nor on levels or other characteristics of exposure. It is, therefore, difficult to select the most appropriate population to study. Excessively large populations would increase the risk of including many subjects with very low exposures thus diluting the effect, if any, while small populations will result in a low number of cases and might include a large proportion of residents employed in the industries under investigation.

Several epidemiological investigations have been performed on lung cancer in industrial areas. Among these may be mentioned the studies by: Blot and Fraumeni [22], indicating a higher lung cancer mortality in areas with chemical, paper and pulp and petroleum industries; Axelsson and Rylander [23], who investigated the possible effects of environmental exposure to chromium due to ferro-chromium alloy industries in Sweden; Shear et al. [24], who analysed one parish in Louisiana which had the highest incidence of lung cancer in the United States and found an increased risk for residents within 1.2 kilometers from industrial facilities; Matanoski

et al. [25], who found an association with arsenical pesticide production facilities.

Iron and steel foundries and non-ferrous smelting plants are the two types of industries most frequently investigated in relation to the potential lung cancer risk resulting from emissions to the environment. Occupational exposure in iron and steel foundries has been shown to increase the risk of lung cancer [26]. Populations residing near iron and steel foundries have been studied particularly in Scotland. In 3 subsequent studies [27-29], researchers from the University of Dundee have investigated the lung cancer mortality in relation to environmental exposure to emissions from iron and steel foundries. The population studied is composed of 3 small communities with old foundries. Following the same methodological approach, the residents in the 3 towns were a priori divided into different subgroups of estimated exposure, based on the soil contamination by metals. In all 3 studies, the highest lung cancer mortality was concentrated in the areas estimated to be more exposed to emissions from the foundries and a decreasing pattern of lung cancer risk was observed with decreasing contamination by metals. The lung cancer excess, which ranged from 30% to 100% in some subgroups, was reduced when adjusted for socioeconomic factors, but the decreasing pattern was not changed.

Possible effects on lung cancer risk from exposure to emissions from non-ferrous smelters have been studied in various countries. Correlation studies have shown an increased lung cancer mortality in relation to residence near non-ferrous smelters [30-33]. A more than 2-fold increase was reported in some of the studies, but the results were inconsistent across the sexes and when adjustment for employment at the smelters was performed. Blot and Fraumeni analysed the U.S. mortality data for the period 1950-69 and found an overall increase in lung cancer rates in 31 counties where non-ferrous smelters were located [34].

Using a case-control approach, Lyon et al. [35], Greaves et al. [36] and Rom et al. [37] tested the association between exposure from non-ferrous smelter emissions and lung cancer risk in 3 smelter counties and failed to demonstrate a relationship between residence and exposure. Two further case-control studies were conducted in the U.S. and Sweden, taking into account the potential confounding from employment at the smelter and smoking. Brown et al. [38] found a 2-fold increased risk of lung cancer associated with residence near a zinc-smelter facility with increased exposure to arsenic, cadmium and several other metals. Similar results were found in a case-control study conducted by Pershagen [39] among men living close to a copper smelter with huge arsenic emissions in northern Sweden. The relative risk for lung cancer among residents in the exposed area was 2.3 for non-smokers and 17.5 for smokers. Considering the RR of 8.3 for smokers in the reference area, the results are suggestive of multiplicative interaction between tobacco smoke and ambient air pollution. Further support of an effect due to exposure to emissions from smelting facilitiles on lung cancer risk comes from a study by Frost et al. [40], who reported an association between lung cancer risk in women living near a U.S. smelter and estimated exposure to airborne arsenic levels.

Overall, the studies suggest that emissions from some types of industries may increase the lung cancer risk of the surrounding population. The evidence is strongest for non-ferrous smelters, where arsenic emissions may be of importance. In addition, increased lung cancer risks have generally been observed among persons employed at these industries, who have been more heavily exposed to the same agents.

Analytical Studies in Urban Populations

Analytical epidemiological studies generally provide the best opportunity to elucidate causal relationships in human populations. Cohort and case-control studies are the two predominant types of such studies. Both these types use individuals as the unit of observation, in the sense that they contain information on exposure(s) and disease(s) of interest for each study subject. As a rule, the case-control design is more effective when rare diseases are studied. On the other hand,

the risks of some types of bias are often greater in case-control than in cohort studies. The available evidence on urban lung cancer risks from *cohort studies* generally comes from studies aimed at investigating risks of tobacco smoking. This implies that data on smoking are often quite extensive, while the exposure information regarding ambient air pollution is less detailed. Most studies did not include any quantitative information on air pollution levels. Furthermore, information on other potential confounders, such as occupational exposures, is limited.

The first major cohort study with data on lung cancer in relation to urban/rural residence included 187,783 white men from 9 U.S. states who were followed from 1952 to 1955 [41]. A total of 11,870 deaths occurred, including 448 from lung cancer. The age and smoking standardised death rate for lung cancer was 75 and 59 per 100,000 man-years in cities of over 50,000 inhabitants and rural areas, respectively, corresponding to a relative death rate of about 1.3. The increased risk was seen both in smokers and non-smokers.

Smoking habits were obtained in 1957 for 69,868 men from the California Division of the American Legion [42]. In the more polluted Los Angeles and San Diego counties, between 0.3% and 6.7% of the maximum hourly oxidant concentrations exceeded 0.15 ppm (300 $\mu g/m^3$) at different locations in 1963. The mortality of the cohort was followed through 1962 and a total of 304 cases of lung cancer were identified. Age- and smoking-adjusted mortality rates for lung cancer were 95.4 per 100,000 man-years in Los Angeles county and 102 per 100,000 in the San Fransisco Bay area and San Diego counties. In other, less urban, Californian counties the corresponding death rate was 75.5 per 100,000, giving a relative death rate in urban areas of about 1.3. The higher relative death rate in urban areas was present both in non-smokers and smokers and an additive effect of urban living and smoking was suggested.

In 1959, more than one million men and women in 25 U.S. states were asked about smoking habits, place of residence, occupational exposures etc. [43]. Over a 6-year follow-up period, 1,510 lung cancer deaths among men were observed. Among men with occupational exposure to "dust, fumes, gases or X-rays" there were age- and smoking-standardised lung cancer death rates of 1.23, 1.14 and 0.98 in metropolitan areas with more than 1 million inhabitants, less than 1 million and non-metropolitan areas, respectively. Corresponding ratios for men without these occupational exposures were 0.98, 0.97 and 0.92, respectively. Data for specific smoking groups were not presented.

In 1963, a sample of 25,444 men and 26,467 women from Sweden responded to a questionnaire on smoking [44]. In a follow-up through 1972, 116 male and 28 female lung cancer cases were observed. For smokers there was a relative lung cancer death rate of about 1.6 in cities (Stockholm, Gothenburg and Malmö) and 1.2 in towns in comparison with rural areas. Too few cases for a meaningful analysis occurred among women and non-smokers. An extended follow up of the male part of the cohort through 1979 showed smoking standardised death rates of 1.4 and 1.1 in cities and towns, respectively (personal communication).

A cohort of 34,440 male British doctors was followed from 1951 to 1971 [45]. Based on residence in 1951, age and smoking-standardised lung cancer death ratios in "conurbations, large towns (50,000-100,000), small towns (<50,000) and rural areas" were calculated at 0.99, 1.07, 0.99 and 0.96, respectively. No information was given on urban/rural rates in different smoking groups.

In a linking of the Swedish National Census in 1960 and the Cancer Registry 1961-1973, a total of 15,799 male and 4,119 female lung cancer cases were identified [46]. Using smoking data available for about 1% of the cohort, Ehrenberg et al. [47] estimated that about 40% and 20% of the lung cancer incidence in males and females, respectively, was "statistically explainable" by urbanisation variables after subtraction of the effects of diagnostic intensity and smoking.

A cohort of 4,475 Finnish men was followed from 1964 to 1980 to study the effects of migration, marital status and smoking as risk factors for cancer [48]. There was a relative risk for lung or laryngeal cancer of about 1.2 for "urbanised" and 0.7 for "urban" smokers in relation to "rural" smokers among married men. The relative risks for unmarried men

and non/past smokers were difficult to interpret because of small numbers.

All *case-control studies* on air pollution and cancer reviewed here contain individual data on smoking, and the most recent studies also include information on occupational exposures. The exposure information for the cases was often obtained from relatives. Data on ambient air levels for different pollutants were generally rather scanty. Most of the studies come from the U.K. and the U.S. and the studies from these countries will be discussed together.

The first study from the U.K. included 725 male lung cancer cases and about 12,000 hospital controls without cancer from North Wales and Liverpool who were identified in the period 1952-1954 [49]. Six-month average concentrations of smoke were reported at between 200 and 350 µg/m^3 in the urban study areas and about 50 µg/m^3 in the rural areas. For benzo(a)pyrene the corresponding levels were between 20 and 80 and about 10 ng/m^3, respectively. There were relative risks of 1.1 to 3.4 in different groups of smokers, when urban and rural areas were compared. An additive effect from urban residence and smoking was suggested.

A series of papers on air pollution and lung cancer in north-east England and Northern Ireland were published by Dean and co-workers [50,51]. Monthly average smoke and sulphur dioxide levels reported from one of the areas in 1972 exceeded 100 µg/m^3. The investigations were of similar design and included from 780 to 2,873 men and from 138 to 199 women who had died of lung cancer. Controls were sampled from the living population of the study areas or among those who died from "non-respiratory illness". The case:control ratio ranged from 1:1 to 1:15. In general, increased lung cancer risks were observed in both men and women in urban areas or areas with "high" levels of air pollution. The age- and smoking-standardised relative risks mostly ranged between 1.5 and 5. Some findings indicated that the combined effects of urban residence and smoking exceeded additivity.

The first 2 case-control studies from the U.S. providing data on urban/rural residence and lung cancer were based on a 10% sample of all white male and female lung cancer deaths in 1958 and 1959 [52,53]. Controls were sampled from the general population. A total of 2,381 male and 749 female cases were included as well as 31,516 male and 34,339 female controls. Overall age- and smoking-standardised mortality ratios of 1.43 and 1.27 were observed in a comparison of urban and rural residence in men and women, respectively. Positive trends in risk with duration of residence were seen for both sexes. In men, the joint effect of smoking and urban residence exceeded additivity, while in women the interaction appeared to be additive.

In Los Angeles county, California, Pike et al. [54] obtained smoking, occupational and residential histories from 1,425 male and 576 female lung cancer cases diagnosed in the period 1972-1975, as well as from 445 male and 186 female population controls. There was an increased lung cancer incidence in "high" air pollution areas in males, which appeared to be fully explained by occupational factors. No association was found between duration of residence in the area and lung cancer risk. Benzo(a)pyrene levels of 3 ng/m³ were reported at the time of the study, but it was estimated that, previously, they were 10 to 20 times higher.

Information on smoking, residence history and occupation was provided by 417 white male lung cancer cases and 752 hospital controls with non-respiratory, non-neoplastic disease admitted to a large hospital in Eire County, New York, between 1957 and 1965 [55]. Two-year average concentrations of total suspended particulates in the early 1960s exceeded 200 μg/m³ in the most heavily polluted areas of the county. Relative risks of about 1.1 and 1.4 for non-smokers and smokers, respectively, were associated with 50 or more years of residence in areas with "high or medium" levels of air pollution. The combined effect of air pollution and smoking appeared to exceed the sum of the 2 exposures.

A population-based study in New Mexico included 283 male and 139 female lung cancer cases as well as 475 population controls identified in the period 1980-1982 [56]. Multiple logistic regression models including smoking, occupation and ethnic group revealed no consistent association of residence history variables with lung cancer risk.

Three further case-control studies on air pollution and lung cancer have been published,

furnishing data from Japan, Poland and China. The Japanese study included 180 male and 79 female lung cancer cases as well as 2,241 male and 2,475 female population controls identified from 1960-1966 in 2 cities near Osaka [57]. Concentrations of suspended matter in 1965 were reported at 190, 220 and 390 μg/m³ in "low, intermediate and high" air pollution areas. Corresponding "maximum" benzo(a)pyrene levels were 26, 31 and 79 ng/m³, respectively. The age- and smoking-adjusted relative risks in areas with "high" levels of air pollution were 1.8 and 1.2 in men and women, respectively, compared with low air pollution areas. The increased risks were primarily seen in smokers.

A study including 901 male and 198 female lung cancer cases, as well as 875 male and 198 female controls with non-respiratory diseases identified from death registers in the period 1980-1985, was performed in the heavily polluted Cracow area in Poland [58]. A combined index of air pollution was used based on total suspended particulates (TSP) and SO_2: Low: TSP <150 μg/m³ and SO_2 <104 μg/m³; medium: TSP >150 μg/m³ or SO_2 >104 μg/m³; high: both TSP and SO_2 above these levels. There was a relative risk of 1.46 for men in high-air pollution areas compared with subjects in low-air pollution areas. A multiplicative interaction was indicated between air pollution, smoking and occupational exposure.

In a population-based study, interviews were performed with 729 male and 520 female lung cancer cases diagnosed 1985-1987 as well as with 788 male and 557 female population controls from Shenyang, China [59]. Ambient air pollution resulted mainly from combustion of coal for home heating and cooking, and from industrial emissions. Monthly average benzo(a)pyrene concentrations of 60 ng/m³ in the winter were reported. Relative risks adjusted for age, education and smoking of 2.3 and 2.5 in men and women, respectively, were found in areas with "smoky" outdoor environment, compared with "non-smoky" areas. Corresponding relative risks were 1.5 and 1.4 in "somewhat/slightly smoky" areas.

In conclusion, it is difficult to interpret the epidemiological evidence on ambient air pollution and lung cancer. Most studies were not originally designed to assess this relation, which has implications for the detail and quality of the exposure information. Data from measurements of air pollutants were generally limited, making it difficult to compare the findings in different studies and to assess dose-response relationships.

It is clear that the environments under study show great differences in the types of exposures. Emissions resulting from the use of coal and other fossil fuels for residential heating were major sources of pollution in some areas, while in others, motor vehicles or industries were more important. It is not possible from the data available to separate effects of residential heating-generated pollutants from those resulting from motor vehicle emissions.

The crude exposure measures used in the epidemiological studies are a major problem. If the imprecision in the exposure assessment is unrelated to the health effects under study, this would lead to underestimation (dilution) of any associations. For example, most of the exposure information provided refers to recent measurements, while the pertinent exposures may have occurred decades ago.

Confounding factors are of great concern in evaluating relative risks of the magnitude encountered in the studies of air pollution and cancer, i.e., in the order of 1.5 or lower. Data on smoking habits were available in most of the analytical studies, but there may still be residual confounding from smoking when urban and rural areas are compared [45]. Occupational exposures may also be important confounders and this was often not controlled in the earlier studies. Other potential confounders in urban/rural comparisons of lung cancer risks include diagnostic intensity [47], dietary habits [60] and domestic radon exposure [61]. It is probable that influences of different confounders vary between the populations under study.

A particular problem affecting the case-control studies is the high mortality of lung cancer. This often resulted in the use of proxy respondents for the cases. However, for the controls exposure information was obtained directly from the study subjects in many of the investigations. It is not clear if this difference in the source of data has resulted in biased estimates of relative risks associated with the exposures.

Other Cancers

Many of the ecological studies discussed earlier in this chapter also included cancers other than lung cancer. Some additional investigations on cancer in urban areas focussed on all sites taken together or on sites other than the respiratory tract [62-65]. Increased total cancer rates in urban areas were often observed, but the relative risks were generally lower than for lung cancer. For specific sites, the results were less consistent.

A few of the analytical epidemiological studies reviewed in the section on lung cancer presented data on urban/rural rates for other sites, controlling for smoking. In the Swedish cohort described by Cederlöf et al. [44], there were positive trends in incidence of bladder cancer in men and cancer of the uterine cervix in women with increasing urbanisation among both non-smokers and smokers. The relative risks were of similar magnitude as those observed for lung cancer.

In the study based on the Utah Cancer Registry described above, increased mortality ratios in urban areas were found for cancer of the oral cavity and pharynx, oesophagus, bladder, colon and prostate among non-Mormon males [21]. The relative risks were often of the same magnitude as for lung cancer, and generally highest for tobacco-related sites. For Mormons, the only increase in urban areas was seen for cancer of the colon. Among women, there was an overall increased cancer risk in urban areas for Mormons, with the most pronounced excess for bladder cancer. In non-Mormons there was a higher risk for cancer of the uterine cervix in urban areas, while the opposite was true for Mormons.

In the Swedish census cohort described by Ehrenberg et al. [47], there was a stronger correlation between degree of urbanisation and total cancer risk in women than in men. Overall, about 25% of the total cancer incidence in both men and women was reported to be "explainable" by factors related to urbanisation other than smoking and diagnostic intensity.

For cancer of all sites, there was a positive trend with increasing residence time in urban areas among married men who were non/past smokers in the Finnish cohort described above [48]. No similar trend was seen among married smokers.

It may be concluded that urban/rural differences in cancer rates are often seen for sites other than the respiratory tract. Even if smoking habits were controlled in some of the studies, residual confounding from smoking is likely to occur. Other factors such as diagnostic intensity, occupational exposures and diet may also have contributed. It is not possible to assess in detail the role of ambient air pollution.

Magnitude of the Effects

The strongest evidence of an effect of air pollution on cancer incidence is seen for lung cancer. Smoking-standardised relative risks comparing urban and rural areas were often in the order of 1.5 or lower in the published studies, and generally higher in men than in women. A relative risk of 1.5 would imply that one-third of the cases among the exposed are "attributable" to the exposure. Corresponding attributable risks for relative risks of 1.1 and 1.3 are 9.1% and 23.1%, respectively. The attributable risk for the whole population is lower and depends on the proportion exposed in the population.

Two of the analytical studies on air pollution and lung cancer provided data on attributable risks (or similar measures). In the national Swedish cohort, Ehrenberg et al. [47] reported that approximately 40% and 20% of the lung cancer incidence in men and women, respectively, were "statistically explainable" by urbanisation variables other than smoking and diagnostic intensity. Smoking explained 85% and 20-40% of the lung cancer incidence in men and women. In the case-control study from the Cracow region, it was estimated that 4.3% of the lung cancers in men and 10.5% in women were attributable to air pollution [58]. Corresponding estimates for smoking and occupational exposure were 74.7% and 20.6% in men, and 47.6% and 8.3% in women.

Cancer risks associated with some of the components of air pollution in urban and in-dustrialised areas have been studied in experimental animals and among occupationally exposed populations. In general, the exposures were of orders of magnitude higher than those encountered in the general environment. Thus, a number of extrapolation models have been proposed, including the generally used non-threshold "average relative risk model" [66].

The WHO recently evaluated cancer risks in humans exposed to various carcinogens in ambient air [1]. Based on extrapolations from epidemiological data on occupational exposures, the lifetime (70-year) lung cancer risk resulting from exposure to 1 $\mu g/m^3$ was estimated at 9×10^{-2} and 4×10^{-3} for benzo(a)pyrene and arsenic, respectively. Assuming a background lifetime risk of lung cancer of 3%, this implies that lifetime exposures of about 170 ng/m^3 of BaP and 4 $\mu g/m^3$ of arsenic are necessary to produce relative risks of the order of 1.5. Levels in this range have earlier been recorded for BaP in cities and for arsenic near copper smelters [1], but are somewhat higher than those reported in the epidemiological studies discussed above. It should be kept in mind, however, that exposure information was only provided in a few of the studies and for a very limited number of agents. Furthermore, the exposure data was often based on recent measurements and earlier levels may have been substantially higher.

After reviewing available experimental and epidemiological evidence, in 1977 a Task Group estimated that "combustion products of fossil fuels in ambient air, probably acting together with cigarette smoke, have been responsible for cases of lung cancer in large urban areas, the numbers produced being of the order of 5-10 cases per 100,000 males per year" [67]. This would correspond to about 10% of the male lung cancer incidence in such cities, and an even lower proportion of the incidence in the smoking part of the population.

Most of the evidence presented in this review indicates that the lung cancer risk attributable to urban residence is higher than the number estimated by the Task Group in 1977. It is not clear, however, how much of this effect can be attributed to air pollution. Recent data suggest that air pollution-related effects in very heavily polluted areas may be at least as great as those indicated by the Task Group. With increasing urbanisation in many countries it is also expected that the population attributable risks related to urban air pollution will grow.

For effects other than lung cancer, the epidemiological evidence in relation to air pollution is less consistent. An overall increase in cancer risk was observed in many studies, and there is room for an effect by air pollution, although other explanations seem more plausible. It is clear from chapter 3 that some systemic distribution of carcinogenic and genotoxic air pollutants and their metabolites takes place among those exposed, which raises the possibility of cancer risks in other organs than the respiratory tract.

Interactions

In several studies on lung cancer aetiology, a multiplicative interaction between smoking and occupational exposures has been observed. Some examples include asbestos [68], arsenic [69] and radon daughters [70]. Multi-stage models for carcinogenesis with agents operating at different stages in the cancer induction process may generate this type of interaction. In other studies, the interaction was less pronounced, more consistent with an additive effect [71,72]. In most studies, it was not possible to conclusively reject either an additive or a multiplicative model, mainly because of a small number of non-smoking lung cancer cases, resulting in a low statistical power of the tests.

The epidemiological studies on urban air pollution and lung cancer gave somewhat inconsistent results as to the type of interaction

with tobacco smoking. Some studies provided evidence of a combined effect exceeding an additive effect, and often compatible with a multiplicative interaction [50,52,55,58]. Other studies were more consistent with an additive effect [42,49,53]. In most of the studies, urban/rural differences in lung cancer rates were more pronounced or only seen among smokers. For example, the study in Utah revealed increased urban rates for non-Mormons only [21]. A positive interaction between urban air pollution and smoking may contribute to these results.

For industrial air pollution and lung cancer, individual data on smoking were obtained only in 2 studies near non-ferrous smelters [38,39]. Interaction was evaluated only in the study by Pershagen and suggested a multiplication of the effects of residence in the smelter area and smoking. This was similar to the interaction between arsenic and smoking observed among workers at the same smelter [69].

The available evidence on ambient air pollution and lung cancer suggests that there may be an interaction with smoking in excess of an additive effect, although the findings are not entirely consistent. The results have to be interpreted with caution, and there may be bias due to both crude exposure measures and uncontrolled confounding. However, the findings are consistent with data on occupational exposures to high doses of some of the agents present in ambient air pollution. In addition, it may be expected that there are interactions between various components of the pollutant mixture in urban and industrial areas, both of synergistic and antagonistic nature. It is not possible to assess the effects of such interactions in detail, but they may help to explain some of the apparently divergent findings in the epidemiological studies.

REFERENCES

1   World Health Organization Regional Office for Europe: Air quality guidelines for Europe. WHO Regional Publications, European Series, Vol 23. Copenhagen 1987

2   Tobacco Research Council, Todd GF (ed) Statistics of Smoking in the United Kingdom. Tobacco Research Council, London 1972

3   Stocks P: Studies on Medical and Population Subjects. Regional and Local Differences in Cancer Death Rates. No 1, HMSO, London 1947

4   Curwen MP, Kennaway EL and Kennaway NM: The incidence of cancer of the lung and larynx in urban and rural districts. Br J Cancer 1954 (8):181-198

5   Hoffman EF and Gilliam AG: Lung cancer mortality. Geographical distribution in the United States for 1948-1949. Publ Health Rep 1954 (69):1033-1042

6   Haenszel W, Marcus SC and Zimmerer EG: Cancer morbidity in urban and rural Iowa. Publ Health Monograph No 37, US Government Printing Office 1956

7   IARC: Cancer Incidence in Five Continents, Vol III. Waterhouse J et al (eds). International Agency for Research on Cancer, Lyon 1976

8   Stocks P: Report on cancer in North Wales and Liverpool region. In: British Empire Cancer Campaign 35th Annual Report 1957. Supplement to Part II - British Empire Cancer Campaign, London 1958

9   Mancuso TF, MacFarlane EM and Porterfield JD: Distribution of cancer mortality in Ohio. Am J Publ Health 1955 (45):58-70

10 Levin ML, Haenszel W, Carroll BE: Cancer incidence in urban and rural areas of New York State. JNCI 1960 (24):1243-1257

11 Goldsmith JR: The "urban factor" in cancer: Smoking, industrial exposures, and air pollution as possible explanations. J Env Pathol Toxicol 1980 (3):205-217

12 Trichopoulos D, Hatzakis A, Wynder E, Katsouyanni K and Kalandidi A: Time trends of tobacco smoking, air pollution, and lung cancer in Athens. Environ Res 1987 (44):169-178

13 IARC: Cancer Incidence in Five Continents, Vol. V. Muir C et al (eds). Publ No 88, International Agency of Research on Cancer, Lyon 1987

14 Royal College of Physicians: Air Pollution and Health. Pitman Medical and Scientific Publishing Co, London 1970

15 Lawther PJ and Waller RE: Trends in urban air pollution in the United Kingdom in relation to lung cancer mortality. Environ Health Perspect 1985 (22):71-73

16 Eastcott DF: The epidemiology of lung cancer in New Zealand. Lancet 1956 (i):37-39

17 Dean G: Lung Cancer among white South Africans. Br Med J 1961 (2):1599-1605

18 Dean G: Lung Cancer in Australia. Med J Aust 1962 (1): 1003- 1011

19 Doll R: Mortality from lung cancer among non-smokers. Br J Cancer 1953 (7):303-312

20 Doll R: Atmospheric pollution and lung cancer. Environ Health Perspect 1978 (22):23-31

21 Lyon JL, Gardner JW and West DW: Cancer risk and life style: Cancer among mormons from 1967-1975. In: Cairns J, Lyon JL and Skonick M (eds) Cancer Incidence in Defined Populations. Banbury Report 4. Cold Spring Harbor Laboratory, New York 1980 pp 3-30

22 Blot WJ and Fraumeni JF: Geographic patterns of lung cancer: Industrial correlation. Am J Epidemiol 1976 (103):539-550

23 Axelsson G and Rylander R: Environmental chromium dust and lung cancer mortality. Environ Res 1980 (23):469-476

24 Shear CL, Seale DB and Gottlieb MS: Evidence for space-time clustering of lung cancer deaths. Environ Health 1980 (35):335-343

25 Matanoski G, Fishbein L, Redmond C, Rosenkranz H and Wallace L: Contribution of organic particulates to respiratory cancer. Environ Health Perspect 1986 (70):37-49

26 IARC: Monographs on the Evaluation of Carcinogenic Risk of Chemicals to Humans, Vol. 34. International Agency for Research on Cancer, Lyon 1984 pp 133-190

27 Lloyd OL: Respiratory cancer clustering associated with localized industrial air pollution. Lancet 1978 (i):318-320

28 Lloyd OL, Smith G, Lloyd MM, Holland Y and Gailey F: Raised mortality from lung cancer and high sex ratios of births associated with industrial pollution. Br J Indust Med 1985 (42):475-480

29 Smith GH, Williams FLR and Lloyd OL: Respiratory cancer and air pollution from iron foundries in a Scottish town: An epidemiological and environmental study. Br J Indust Med 1987 (44):795-802

30 Newman JA, Saccomanno G, Auerbach O, Archer V, Kuschner M Grondahl R and Wilson J: Histologic types of bronchogenic carcinoma among members of copper-mining and smelting communities. Ann N Y Acad Sci 1975 (271):250-268

31 Pershagen G, Elinder CG and Bolander AM: Mortality in a region surrounding an arsenic emitting plant. Environ Health Perspect 1977 (19):133-137

32 Cordier S, Theriault G and Iturra H: Mortality patterns in a population living near a copper smelter. Environ Res 1983 (31):311-322

33 Xiao HP and Xu ZY: Air pollution and lung cancer in Liaoning Province, People's Republic of China. NCI Monogr 1985 (69):53-58

34 Blot WJ and Fraumeni JF: Arsenical air pollution and lung cancer. Lancet 1975 (22):142-144

35 Lyon J, Filmore JL and Klauber MR: Arsenical air pollution and lung cancer. Lancet 1977 (22):869

36 Greaves WW, Rom WN, Lyon JL, Varley G, Wright DD and Chiu G: Relationship between lung cancer and distance of residences from nonferrous smelter stack effluent. Am J Indust Med 1981 (2):15-23

37 Rom WN, Varley G, Lyon JL and Shopkow S: Lung cancer mortality among residents living near the El Paso smelter. Br J Indust Med 1982 (39):269-272

38 Brown LM, Pottern LM and Blot WJ: Lung cancer in relation to environmental pollutants emitted from industrial sources. Environ Res 1984 (34):250-261

39 Pershagen, G: Lung cancer mortality among men living near an arsenic-emitting smelter. Am J Epidemiol 1985 (122):684-694

40 Frost F, Hfarter L, Milham S, Royce R, Smith A, Hartley J and Enterline P: Lung cancer among women residing close to an arsenic emitting copper smelter. Arch Environ Health 1987 (42):471-475

41 Hammond EC and Horn D: Smoking and death rates - report on fortyfour months of follow-up of 187783 men. J Am Med Assoc 1958 (166):1294-1308

42 Buell P, Dunn JE and Breslow L: Cancer of the lung and Los Angeles type air pollution. Cancer 1967 (20):2139-2147

43 Hammond EC: Smoking habits and air pollution in relation to lung cancer. In: Lee DHK (ed) Environmental factors in respiratory disease. Academic Press, New York 1972 pp 177-198

44 Cederlöf R, Friberg L, Hrubec Z and Lorich U: The relationship of smoking and some social covariables to mortality and cancer morbidity. Department of Environmental Hygiene, Karolinska Institutet, Stockholm 1975

45 Doll R and Peto R: The causes of cancer: Quantitative estimates of avoidable risks of cancer in the United States today. JNCI 1981 (66):1191-1308

46 The Swedish Cancer-Environment Registry 1961-1973. National Board of Health and Welfare, Stockholm 1980

47 Ehrenberg L, von Bahr B and Ekman G: Register analysis of measures of urbanization and cancer incidence in Sweden. Environ Internat 1985 (11):393-399

48 Tenkanen L and Teppo L: Migration, marital status and smoking as risk determinants of cancer. Scand J Soc Med 1987 (15): 67-72

49 Stocks P and Campbell J: Lung cancer death rates among nonsmokers and pipe and cigarette smokers. Br Med J 1955 (2):923-929

50 Dean G: Lung cancer and bronchitis in Northern Ireland. Br Med J 1966 (1):1506-1514

51 Dean G, Lee PN, Todd GF and Wicken AJ: Report on a second retrospective mortality study in North-East England. Part 1 & 2. Tobacco Research Council, London 1977 & 1978

52 Haenszel W, Loveland DB and Sirken MG: Lung-cancer mortality as related to residence and smoking histories: White males. JNCI 1962 (28):947-1001

53 Haenszel W and Taeuber KE: Lung-cancer mortality as related to residence and smoking histories: White females. JNCI 1964 (32):803-838

54 Pike MC, Jing JS, Rosario IP, Henderson BE and Menck HR: Occupation: Explanation of an apparent air pollution related localized excess of lung cancer in Los Angeles County. In: Breslow L and Whittemore A (eds) Energy and Health. SIAM-SIMS Conference series, Philadelphia 1979 pp 3-16

55 Vena JE: Air pollution as a risk factor in lung cancer. Am J Epidemiol 1982 (116):42-56

56 Samet JM, Humble CG, Skipper BE and Pathak DR: History of residence and lung cancer risk in New Mexico. Am J Epidemiol 1987 (125):800-811

57 Hitosugi M: Epidemiological study of lung cancer with special reference to the effect of air pollution and smoking habit. Bull Inst Publ Health 1968 (17):236-255

58 Jedrychowski W, Becher H, Wahrendorf J and Basa-Cierpialek Z: A case-control study of lung cancer with special reference to the effect of air pollution in Poland. J Epidemiol Commun Health 1990 (in press)

59 Xu ZY, Blot WJ, Xiao HP, Wu A, Feng YP, Stone BJ, Jie S, Ershow AG, Henderson BE and Fraumeni JF: Smoking, air pollution and the high rates of lung cancer in Shenyang, China. JNCI 1989 (8):1800-1806

60 Jedrychowski W, Wahrendorf J, Popiela T and Rachtan J: A case-control study of dietary factors and stomach cancer risk in Poland. Int J Cancer 1986 (37):837-842

61 Svensson C, Pershagen G and Klominek J: Lung cancer in women and type of dwelling in relation to radon exposure. Cancer Res 1989 (49): 1861-1865

62 Winkelstein W and Kantor S: Stomach cancer: Positive association with suspended particulate air pollution. Arch Environ Health 1969 (18):544-547

63 Demopoulos HB and Gutman EG: Cancer in New Jersey and other complex urban/industrial areas. J Environ Path Toxicol 1980 (3):219-235

64 Robertson LS: Environmental correlates of intercity variation in age-adjusted cancer mortality rates. Environ Health Perspect 1980 (36):197-203

65 Blondell JM: Urban-rural factors affecting cancer mortality in Kentucky, 1950-1969. Cancer Det Prev 1988 (11):209-223

66 EPA. Health assessment document for acrylonitrile. US Environmental Protection Agency, Washington, DC 1983

67 Cederlöf, R, Doll R, Fowler B, Friberg L, Nelson N and Vouk V: Air pollution and cancer: Risk assessment methodology and epidemiologic evidence. Report of a Task Group. Environ Health Perspect 1978 (22):2-10

68 Hammond EC, Selikoff IJ and Seidman H: Asbestos exposure, cigarette smoking and death rates. Ann NY Acad Sci 1979 (330):473-496

69 Pershagen G, Wall S, Taube A and Linnman L: On the interaction between occupational arsenic exposure and smoking and its relationship to lung cancer. Scand J Work Environ Health 1981 (7):302-309

70 Archer VE, Wagoner JK and Lundin FE: Uranium mining and cigarette smoking effects on man. J Occup Med 1973 (15):204-211

71 Pinto SS, Henderson V and Enterline PE: Mortality experience of arsenic exposed workers. Arch Environ Health 1978 (33):325-331

72 Radford EP and St Clair-Renard KG: Lung cancer in Swedish iron miners exposed to low doses of radon daughters. N Engl J Med 1984 (310):1485-1494

Cancer Risk Estimation and Prevention

John D. Graham

Associate Professor of Policy and Decision Sciences, Department of Health Policy and Management, Harvard School of Public Health, 677 Huntington Ave., Boston, MA 02115, U.S.A.

Since scientific evidence suggests that human exposure to outdoor air pollution may increase the incidence of cancer, it is prudent for decision makers to investigate the magnitude of the potential problem and adapt feasible prevention strategies. In this chapter, we use a "risk analysis/risk management" framework to examine prevention opportunities. Our objective is to show how environmental science and economics can be utilised together to inform the development of prevention policies. Throughout the chapter, we highlight the difficulties associated with implementing a risk analysis/risk management approach, given our current state of scientific knowledge about air pollution and human health.

The chapter begins with a discussion of how scientific data are used to make quantitative estimates of cancer risk due to exposure to outdoor air pollutants. Although such estimates can be useful in targeting the major sources of pollution-induced cancer, the chapter highlights the assumptions and uncertainties associated with current tools of risk estimation. The chapter then discusses a variety of technical strategies that decision makers can employ to prevent outdoor air pollution. We emphasise how the economics of fossil fuels play an important role in the success or failure of many control strategies. Finally, the chapter illustrates how cost-effectiveness analysis can be used by decision makers to inform the choice among alternative prevention policies. Examples are described for the control of both mobile and stationary sources of air pollution.

Risk Estimation

Quantitative estimates of excess cancer risk due to outdoor air pollution are potentially useful in targeting priorities for prevention. In theory, risk estimates can provide an objective basis for deciding which sources or pollutants are most important and which are relatively trivial. Since decision makers have limited resources to invest in prevention, information about the magnitudes of various cancer risks can be quite useful.

Unfortunately, the challenge of making accurate cancer risk estimates for air pollutants is formidable, due to gaps in scientific knowledge. Scientists do not know how much human cancer is caused by outdoor air pollution, although attempts have been made to make some rough estimates [1-3]. Despite the scientific obstacles, the U.S. Environmental Protection Agency has developed a standard procedure for making cancer risk estimates that is now in widespread use [4]. The procedure has the advantage of making use of the growing body of scientific data that is available for specific pollutants. Such data may address emission rates, patterns of atmospheric dispersion and transformation, levels of human exposure, toxicity, carcinogenicity and epidemiology. As we shall see, the scientific basis of the EPA procedure is still somewhat shaky and needs to be improved, where possible, by incorporating scientific information about pharmacokinetics and mechanism of action.

Before describing the EPA approach, it is important to recognise that any method of risk estimation for outdoor air pollutants must use assumptions or models at two critical stages.

Firstly, the method must embody a procedure for extrapolating responses observed in animals to responses that may occur in humans. For most pollutants, we lack direct information on how the incidence of human cancer is affected by outdoor air pollution. Secondly, the method must embody a procedure for extrapolating responses at high doses to responses that may occur at low doses. Whether the original dose-response data come from animals or humans, the responses will inevitably be at levels of exposure that are far above the levels observed in the typical outdoor environment. In light of these inherent uncertainties in risk estimation, EPA has designed a method that is intended to produce a plausible upper bound on excess cancer risk due to air pollution. That is, the EPA procedure is designed to produce a risk estimate for each exposure scenario that is unlikely to understate the true (yet unknown) risk.

EPA recently examined how much cancer incidence in the U.S.A. may be attributable to 90 "toxic" air pollutants emitted from 60 source categories [5,6]. The list of pollutants does not include the more ubiquitous pollutants (ozone, lead, sulphur dioxide, carbon monoxide, nitrogen dioxide and particulates) that EPA regulates through a special process. Nor does the list include hundreds of other airborne chemicals that have not been adequately studied from the standpoint of toxicity or human exposure. The report was intended as a "scoping" study to determine what level of regulatory priority the U.S. should give to carcinogenic air pollutants.

Before describing the findings of the EPA report, we shall scrutinise how risk estimates were developed for two specific air pollutants, benzene and formaldehyde. Benzene serves to illustrate how occupational epidemiology is used in risk estimation, while formaldehyde illustrates how data from long-term rodent bioassays are used in risk estimation.

Although we shall focus our attention on uncertainties in the evaluation of dose-response relationships, the reader should also be aware that the exposure information used by EPA depends primarily on the use of emission, dispersion and exposure models. In some cases, ambient measurements of pollutant concentrations are used. Only rarely are data available from personal exposure monitoring. Moreover, EPA's exposure models do not usually incorporate information about how much of the inhaled pollutant (or its toxic metabolites) is actually delivered to target cells in the body. This kind of pharmacokinetic information in humans is rare and is available for relatively few air pollutants.

Benzene

EPA's national risk estimate for benzene (181 cases of cancer per year in the U.S.A.) is based on average measured concentrations of 8 micrograms per cubic metre for urban populations and 0.6 micrograms per cubic metre for rural populations. Using relative risk estimates obtained from occupational epidemiology, EPA predicts that 70 years of exposure to 1 microgram per cubic metre of benzene will increase a person's risk of cancer by as much as 8.3 in a million - or one year of exposure will (theoretically) increase risk by as much as 0.119 in a million. Hence, the 185 million urban Americans are estimated to experience 176 benzene-induced cancers each year, while the 70 million rural Americans are estimated to experience 5 benzene-induced cancers each year.

The key number in this calculation, the "unit risk factor" of 8.3 in a million, is an extrapolation of the excess incidence of leukaemia documented among workers exposed to relatively high and intermittent concentrations of benzene. Although several epidemiological studies of workers have demonstrated that benzene exposure is associated with an excess risk of leukaemia [7-9], EPA's risk estimates for benzene rely primarily on a particular study sponsored by the National Institute of Occupational Safety and Health (NIOSH).

The NIOSH study reported on a cohort of 1,165 white male workers exposed to benzene after World War II in two rubber hydrochloride (Pliofilm) manufacturing plants, one in Akron, Ohio and the other in St. Mary's, Ohio [10]. They found a total of 9 leukaemia deaths, compared to 2.7 expected (based on the mortality experience of the general U.S. white male population) - or a crude relative risk (RR) of 3.3. Retrospective exposure assessment suggests a dose-response relationship. The RRs were 1.09 for workers with less than 40 ppm-years of cumulative exposure, 3.22 for workers with between 40 and 200 ppm-years of cumulative exposure, 11.86 with between 200 and 400 ppm-years of exposure, and 66.37 with 400 or more ppm-years of exposure. By way of comparison, the average urban American dweller is exposed to 0.02642 ppm benzene in outdoor air, or 1.8 ppm years of benzene exposure for 70 years of urban living.

The validity of EPA's risk estimate for benzene has been questioned on numerous grounds.

Firstly, some observers have cautioned against using epidemiological data in risk estimation when a small number of cases determine the relative risk estimates and when exposure information is sketchy [11]. Note that the RRs in the NIOSH study are based on 9 cases of leukaemia. Moreover, the exposure assessment for the NIOSH cohort involves a considerable amount of guesswork.

Secondly, cumulative exposure to benzene may not be the biologically correct measure of exposure. In particular, recent laboratory evidence indicates that intermittent exposure to benzene is more toxic than continuous exposure, holding constant the amount of cumulative exposure [12,13]. The timing pattern of exposure appears to be at least as important as the absolute amount of benzene administered in generating toxic and carcinogenic responses. Since the workers in the NIOSH cohort were exposed to benzene intermittently, their responses may not be relevant to people who breathe low levels of benzene continuously throughout a lifetime.

Finally, even if cumulative exposure to benzene is a biologically relevant measure of exposure, it does not necessarily follow that cancer risk is proportional to cumulative exposure at low exposure levels. Statisticians have arrived at conflicting conclusions about which dose-response models are appropriate in the case of benzene [14]. Although the hypothesis of a no-effect level cannot be proven or refuted with available data, some scientists believe that bone marrow toxicity is a necessary precursor to benzene-induced leukaemia [15].

Formaldehyde

EPA's national risk estimate for formaldehyde (128 cases of cancer per year in the U.S.A.) is based on average outdoor urban concentrations of 3.16 micrograms per cubic metre and average rural concentrations of 1.50 micrograms per cubic metre. These figures are based on recent ambient measurements that are somewhat larger than the earlier EPA figures that had been based on modelling exercises.

EPA predicts that 70 years of exposure to 1 microgram per cubic metre of formaldehyde will increase a person's risk of cancer by 1.3 in 100,000. This unit risk factor is based on the malignant tumour incidence data from the Chemical Industry Institute of Toxicology's long-term rodent bioassay of formaldehyde. (Note that this unit risk factor is about 36% larger than the unit risk factor for benzene.) Given the urban-rural distribution of the U.S. population, EPA predicts that outdoor formaldehyde concentrations are responsible for as many as 109 cases of cancer per year among urban residents and 19 cases of cancer per year among rural residents.

EPA's unit risk factor for formaldehyde is derived from CIIT's long-term inhalation bioassay, which administered formaldehyde to Fischer 344 rats and B6C3F1 mice of both sexes at concentrations of 0, 2, 6 and 15 ppm for 24 months. The incidence of squamous cell carcinomas of the nasal cavity in rats was 0% among controls (0/208), 0% at 2 ppm (0/210), 1% at 6 ppm (2/210), and 50% (103/206) at 15 ppm [16]. Note that the 2.5-fold increase in administered concentration (from 6 to 15 ppm) was associated with a 50-fold increase in the incidence of malignant tumours (1% to 50%). The results in the mice were less dramatic, since the only positive response occurred in the highest exposure group (0%, 0%, 0%, 3.3%, respectively in the 4 exposure groups). EPA used the rat data for purposes of risk estimation.

The unit risk factor is obtained by fitting the rat data to a linearised version of the multistage model. This model, which is now widely accessible through computer software, is a restricted version of the multistage model that compels a linear dose-response relationship at sufficiently low doses. The slope of the dose-response line at low doses is the largest value that does not flunk a statistical test of compatibility with the experimental responses. Thus, while CIIT's cancer incidence data for rats are highly non-linear within the experimental range, the linearised multistage model is still used by EPA to extrapolate carcinogenic risk to exposure levels below the experimental range.

For an intuitive feel of how this procedure works, note first that EPA's unit risk factor of 1.3 in 100,000 for 70 years of exposure to 1 microgram per cubic metre formaldehyde can be expressed as 1.2 in 100,000 for 70 years of exposure to 1 part per billion formaldehyde. Next, recall that a lifetime of exposure to 6 parts per million formaldehyde caused a cancer incidence of roughly 1% among the rats in the CIIT study. Employing a linear extrapolation to 1 part per billion from the incidence observed at 6 ppm, we divide 0.01 by 6,000 and obtain a risk of 1.7 in a million for a lifetime exposure to 1 part per billion formaldehyde.

In this case, the linear extrapolation places us within an order of magnitude of the estimate produced by the linearised multistage model. More precisely, EPA's unit risk estimate is about a factor of 7 larger than would result from a simple linear extrapolation of the cancer incidence observed in rats at 6 ppm. Our linear extrapolation would have performed even better as an approximation of EPA's procedure if, instead of using the observed incidence of 1% at 6 ppm, we had used the upper confidence limit on the incidence of cancer observed at 6 ppm. This adjustment would account for the fact that the 1% incidence figure is based on a sample of only 210 rats. Due to sampling error, it is possible that the observed incidence in an infinite sample of rats would be as high as 3% to 4%. Using the 4% figure as an upper bound on the "true" incidence of cancer at 6 ppm, we can make a simple linear extrapolation that comes within a factor of 2 of the unit risk factor used by EPA for a lifetime exposure to 1 part per billion. More rigorous discussions of the linearised multistage model are available elsewhere [17].

As we saw in the case of benzene, serious criticisms are levelled against such attempts at quantitative risk estimation. The major criticisms of EPA's formaldehyde risk estimate are summarised below. In light of some of these criticisms and new data, EPA is now reexamining its assessment of formaldehyde.

Firstly, some scientists believe that it is premature to quantify human cancer risk at low exposure levels on the basis of carcinogenic responses observed in rodents at relatively high exposure levels. This reservation applies not just to formaldehyde but to several hundred chemicals that have tested positive in long-term rodent bioassays. These scientists argue that our scientific understanding of chemical carcinogenesis is too primitive to permit reliable quantitative risk estimation. Our ability to accurately extrapolate responses across species is particularly limited [18].

Secondly, new biological data on formaldehyde seem to indicate that the amount of formaldehyde delivered to target cells in rats and monkeys vanishes as the concentrations of formaldehyde administered to animals decline. This non-linear relationship between delivered and administered doses suggests that EPA's unit risk estimate of formaldehyde overstates risk by several orders of magnitude at exposure levels in the part per billion range [19-20].

Thirdly, some scientists believe that EPA should depart from its standard linearised multistage model in the case of formaldehyde, due to the non-linear shape of the experimental data and the known role that cell proliferation plays in the chemical's toxicity. An alternative approach, which is to rely on the maximum likelihood estimate of the multistage model, would retain the non-threshold assumption but predict a non-linear relationship between exposure and cancer incidence at low exposure levels [17,21].

Fourthly, some scientists have criticised EPA for not including benign tumours (polypoid adenomas) and various precursor lesions in the quantitative risk estimate of formaldehyde. Although the CIIT investigators found no evidence that these tumours progress into squamous cell carcinomas, it is possible that a fraction of them progress into adenocarcinomas. If a fraction of the benign tumours were added to the carcinomas to obtain an overall tumour incidence rate, then EPA's unit risk factor would be larger than it is currently estimated to be [22].

Finally, scientists have reached divergent conclusions about how to interpret the growing body of epidemiological data on formaldehyde. Some interpret the results as providing limited evidence of carcinogenicity in humans, others see the results as negative, and others believe that the human data are uninterpretable. In any event, none of the epidemiological studies have the requisite statistical power to refute or confirm EPA's unit risk estimate for exposure levels in the part per billion range [11].

Overall EPA Findings

EPA added the risk estimates for 90 pollutants at 60 source categories to obtain a national estimate of cancer incidence due to outdoor air pollution. Their overall estimate is 1,700 to 2,700 excess cases of cancer per year in the U.S.A., or an equivalent of roughly 7 to 11 annual cases of cancer per million population. The authors of the report emphasise that their estimates are not necessarily appropriate as absolute predictions and are intended to be used for comparison purposes.

The largest single source of excess cancer incidence was motor vehicles, which accounted for 58% of total estimated incidence. Large industrial facilities ("point sources") accounted for another 20% of the estimated national incidence, while small diffuse facilities such as wood stoves and dry cleaners accounted for the remaining incidence (22%). The 7 pollutants estimated to be responsible for more than 100 annual cases of cancer were benzene, 1,3-Butadiene, chloroform, chromium (hexavalent), dioxin, formaldehyde and products of incomplete combustion.

Our examination of the risk estimates for benzene and formaldehyde indicates that these numbers must be treated with caution, even for comparative purposes. For example, if the risk estimates for benzene and formaldehyde are substantially overstated, then motor vehicles might not be as important a source as these numbers suggest. As the scientific basis of risk estimation improves, such numbers can be used by decision makers with a greater degree of confidence.

Prevention Opportunities

Although cancer is only one of many potential adverse consequences of outdoor air pollution, the risk of cancer may spur decision makers to explore strategies for reducing air pollution. Selection of appropriate strategies will generally depend in part on which emission control measures are technically and economically feasible for particular sources. In this section, we discuss briefly various pollution control strategies that decision makers may want to consider. Insofar as air pollution is a significant cause of human cancer, public health professionals would regard these strategies as primary disease prevention policies.

The addition of emission control equipment to stationary and mobile sources of air pollution can result in sharp reductions in the rate of air emissions compared to uncontrolled emission conditions. For example, such equipment has been quite effective in reducing emissions from motor vehicles and electric utilities. Once such equipment is installed, monitoring and maintenance of emission control performance is usually critical to achieving sustained pollution control. While add-on equipment is well-suited for end-of-stack or exhaust pipe emissions, it is not necessarily effective at reducing various fugitive emissions from the numerous doors, cracks, and leaks present at many production facilities. Such add-on equipment can rarely eliminate the emission problem and may create some new problems of waste disposal. In the long run, economic growth and the increase in the number of pollution sources can outstrip the reductions in emissions that are achieved by add-on equipment.

Innovation in the design of industrial and combustion processes promises more effective emission control than can be achieved by add-on equipment. For example, it is unlikely that fugitive emissions at coke plants throughout the world can be reduced to acceptable levels solely through the addition of add-on emission control equipment. Research and development into new steel-making processes that do not require coke production is environmentally attractive. However, such a radical reform of steel making is not yet technically and economically feasible and may take decades to become reality [23]. One of the benefits of applying stringent air-quality-control requirements to industrial processes is that they can spur research and development into the design of cleaner industrial processes.

Since combustion of fossil fuels (coal and oil particularly) is a major source of air pollution, the development of clean, alternative energy sources must be considered an attractive pollution control strategy. The most feasible alternative today is nuclear power, although its public acceptance varies throughout the world. Solar energy and wind power offer some promise as sources of electricity but are not yet economically competitive in many regions of the world. Natural gas is perhaps the cleanest source of energy and its use is rapidly increasing. The use of ethanol or methanol as a fuel for motor vehicles is beginning to receive more serious consideration in the United States, although these fuels may create some air toxic problems of their own that need to be controlled. As long as world oil prices remain relatively depressed, it will be difficult for alternative energy sources to capture increasing shares of the energy market.

Energy conservation is another promising approach to air pollution control that is not utilised adequately in the residential, industrial and transportation sectors of the world economy. In the United States, for example, many highly polluted urban areas have weak mass transit systems and little encouragement for car pooling arrangements during commuting hours. While the high and unstable oil prices of the 1970s spurred some efforts at energy conservation, the return to relatively cheap oil in the 1980s has undercut the economic incentive for energy conservation. Several countries in Europe encourage conservation through taxes and fees on petrol consumption.

Like energy conservation, recycling of materials and waste offers significant promise as a pollution prevention strategy. The recycling of cans, bottles and paper, for example, has become a significant industry in many parts of the world that prevents air pollution which would otherwise occur at production facilities. Separation and recycling of solid waste can also reduce the need for construction of new waste incineration capacity, which is increasingly recognised as a potential source of toxic air emissions [24].

In order to stimulate the prevention or reduction of air pollution, decision makers need to recognise air pollution as a public health problem and utilise policy instruments that encourage pollution control. In the United States, command-and-control regulation in the form of detailed emission limits or technology requirements for each source has been the most widely used policy instrument for the last 20 years. The results have been mixed, and many environmentalists are turning to economic incentives or penalties as an alternative approach to curbing air pollution. Taxes or fees on emissions need to be used more widely to discourage emissions and encourage research and development into innovative pollution control methods [25]. Without a significant change in the economics of fossil fuel consumption, it is doubtful that dramatic progress against air pollution will be made in the foreseeable future.

Cost-Effective Prevention

The control of air pollution can be quite costly. Economists have estimated that the total costs of existing air pollution control programmes in the United States are about $35 billion per year - $15 billion for mobile sources and $20 billion for stationary sources [26]. These cost estimates account for depreciated capital expenditures, operating and maintenance expenditures and a variety of indirect costs such as reduced productivity and innovation. If the Bush Administration's new clean air proposal is enacted into law, these annual costs could increase by 50% or more by the mid-1990s.

Although comparable cost estimates for pollution control are not available on a global basis, it is possible to obtain global information on one significant component of this cost: annual expenditures for new air pollution control equipment. The firm Temple, Barker and Sloane, Inc. has estimated that global expenditures for new air pollution control equipment will approach $5.3 billion in 1989 [27]. These expenditures are divided among Europe (45%), the United States (25%), Japan (15%) and all other nations (15%). As a percentage of Gross National Product, pollution control expenditures in Canada and the United States are smaller than they are in West Germany and Japan.

In light of the substantial costs of pollution control programmes, it is important that such programmes be subjected to cost-effectiveness analysis (CEA). The purpose of CEA is to determine whether programmes are achieving air quality goals at minimum cost or, alternatively, whether fixed investments in pollution control are being allocated in a manner that maximises air quality improvement [28]. To measure programme effectiveness, analysts use either estimates of how much pollution will be removed (e.g., in tons) or estimates of how many cases of cancer will be prevented (which requires quantitative risk estimates). For illustrative purposes, we shall describe several such analyses below.

Controlling Emissions from Motor Vehicles

In most regions of the world, motor vehicles are a significant source of air pollution. Since stationary and mobile sources emit many of the same pollutants, a critical question becomes which sources can be controlled in the most cost-effective fashion. The answer to this question will vary among nations and over time due to differences in technology and incremental estimates of cost and emission control effectiveness.

In the United States, economists have estimated the incremental cost of controlling hydrocarbons, carbon monoxide and nitrogen dioxide from stationary and mobile sources. They have determined that the marginal cost of removing an extra ton of pollution from motor vehicles through design change has been greater than the marginal cost of reducing the same amount of pollution from various stationary sources. For example, the estimated marginal cost per ton of emissions reduced for America's 1981 new car emission standards was about $400 - or more than twice as large as the cost per ton of removing the same pollutants from stationary sources ($160 per ton) [29]. Interestingly, these cost-effectiveness comparisons have not deterred American policy makers from requiring progressively stricter exhaust pipe emission standards for new cars. The U.S. Congress is considering new vehicle emission standards for the mid-1990s that transcend the current

technological capabilities of vehicle and engine manufacturers.

Unless the use of motor vehicles can be curtailed significantly, emissions must be reduced by curtailing the amount of pollution emitted from the exhaust pipe. Economists have also compared the cost-effectiveness of two different strategies for achieving this goal: tightening new vehicle emission standards or requiring states to implement motor vehicle inspection and maintenance programmes. The latter policy can, in principle, address all vehicles on the road while the former policy must operate gradually as cleaner new vehicles replace dirty old vehicles.

The results of this CEA are, again, likely to vary from nation to nation due to differences in baseline levels of emissions from new and old vehicles and differences in the incremental costs and effectiveness of the two policies under consideration. In the United States, the basic finding has been that the cost per ton of emission reduction is lower for stringent inspection and maintenance than for tighter new vehicle emission standards [29]. The difficulty with this comparison is that one of the unmeasured costs of inspection/maintenance, the inconvenience to vehicle owners, has a high degree of salience among America's elected politicians. Thus, America continues to require ever more stringent new vehicle emission standards, even though emission control performance deteriorates as vehicles age since motorists do not maintain the equipment. This problem explains in part the motivation behind proposals to convert motor vehicles from petrol to alternative fuels such as methanol.

In addition to exhaust pollution, motor vehicles also emit pollution during the process of refuelling petrol tanks. Refuelling emissions, which are volatile organic compounds, are a contributor to the smog problem and may increase the incidence of cancer among people who inhale the vapours. The control options include: (1) require petrol stations to "control at the pump" through installation of Stage II vapour recovery systems; and (2) require vehicle manufacturers to redesign fuel tanks with "on-board canisters" that capture petrol vapours and reuse them.

The cost-effectiveness analyses of this question have not reached a definitive conclusion but they have shed light on the key decision

factors [30]. Taking into account both estimated emission control effectiveness and the
costs of new equipment and maintenance, it
appears that control at the pump is more cost
effective (i.e., lower cost per unit of emission
control) than the on-board canisters.
Moreover, controls at the pump can be applied selectively in geographical areas where
the smog problem is particularly serious.

In the final analysis, the potential cancer risks
from inhaling petrol vapours become an important decision factor, because a serious
cancer threat would tilt the analysis in favour
of the more expensive on-board canister
since it is more effective. If, however, smog
control is the only anticipated health benefit,
then the analysis tends to favour controls at
the pump in those regions of the world with
severe smog problems. Unfortunately, the
existing scientific evidence on the potential
carcinogenic risks of inhaling unleaded petrol
vapours is not adequate to make reliable estimates of the human risk [31]. In light of the
scientific uncertainties, the decision has become politicised in the United States and the
ultimate resolution is not yet apparent.

The example of refuelling emissions illustrates that while cost-effectiveness analysis
can offer insight into the choice of prevention
strategies, the analytical tool cannot substi-
tute for a lack of scientific understanding of
the relationship between air pollution and
human cancer. In this respect, the measures
of effectiveness used by economists are often
dependent on the scientific underpinnings of
cancer risk estimates.

Controlling Emissions from Stationary Sources

In controlling emissions from major industrial
facilities, cost-effectiveness analysis has
played an important role in identifying which
emissions within industry can be prevented
most cheaply. For example, reducing emissions from smokestacks through process
changes and add-on equipment has generally been less expensive than reducing fugitive emissions from leaks, valves and doors
[23]. Nor are the costs of emission control uniform across plants within the same firm or
across firms within the same industry. Factors
such as the age of a plant, its original design

and upkeep, and operating practices can influence the marginal costs of emission control.

In light of the above considerations,
economists have shown that it is not necessarily cost effective for regulators to try to
specify a uniform level of pollution control for
firms within an industry or even for all plants
within a single firm. Since the marginal costs
of emission control may vary among plants
and firms, it is less expensive to achieve any
specified emission control objective by allow-
ing some firms/plants to emit more pollution
than others. Although such an approach
might seem inequitable, it can offer enormous
reductions in the overall cost of pollution control.

Rather than require each emission source at
a plant to be controlled through specified
methods, EPA has begun to use plantwide
standards ("bubbles") that allow plant managers to identify and implement the most cost-
effective methods of emission control. In the
iron and steel and petrochemical industries,
the use of plantwide standards has resulted
in a 20% reduction in the cost of emission
control compared to source-specific standards. Even larger savings have been identified in the chemical industry if corporate
managers are permitted to trade emissions
among plants [26]. Such "trading" schemes
allow companies to continue emissions at
plants with large marginal costs of control if
less costly emission reductions can be ac-
complished at plants that have already satis-
fied source-specific standards.

The same concepts of cost-effectiveness can
be implemented on an industry-wide basis by
permitting firms to buy and sell the permission
to pollute. Rather than achieve an industry-
wide emission goal through plant-specific
standards, the government might sell the
rights to pollute to firms and allow these rights
to be bought and sold in a competitive market. Under such a pollution-rights scheme,
firms with relatively large marginal costs of
emission control would buy pollution rights
from firms that find it relatively cheaper to
curtail their emissions. The government can
control the total amount of emissions from the
industry by restricting the number of permits
that are available for sale. In the final analysis, each firm compares the cost of buying an

emission permit to the cost of emission control.

One of the difficulties with both "bubble" and "trading" policies occurs when companies would prefer to control pollutant A rather than pollutant B. Unless both pollutants are of equal carcinogenic potency, it does not necessarily make sense to allow such flexibility in the emission control process. Moreover, the same pollutant may be easier to control at plant A than at plant B, but the population densities around the two plants may not be equivalent. Hence, cost-effectiveness considerations must be pursued with an understanding of the ultimate implications for public health. Once again, these implications can be known only as the scientific basis of risk estimation improves in the future.

Conclusion

Reducing human exposure to air pollution promises significant public health, ecological and economic benefits. In this chapter, we examined only one type of benefit: reduced risk of cancer. Quantifying the excess risk of cancer due to air pollution is fraught with uncertainty, but risk estimates should become more reliable as scientific knowledge advances. In the interim, decision makers should recognise the fragility of the current estimates of human cancer risk due to air pollution. Despite their limitations, such estimates can be used by decision makers to help set priorities for pollution prevention efforts.

The chapter highlighted a variety of strategies for reducing human exposure to air pollution. Dramatic progress will probably not occur until the relative price of fossil fuel consumption - a major source of pollution - increases substantially throughout the world. Nonetheless, modest progress toward cleanup throughout can be made by directly controlling emissions from motor vehicles and factories.

Since pollution control is often costly and resources are limited, decision makers should examine the relative costs and effectiveness of alternative pollution control strategies. The method of cost-effectiveness analysis can assist decision makers in using resources wisely. Policy tools such as emission fees and marketable emission permits can be used to enhance the cost-effectiveness of pollution control programmes. Such tools must, however, be implemented in a fashion that does not compromise the achievement of public health objectives.

REFERENCES

1   Doll R and Peto R: The causes of cancer: Quantitative estimates of avoidable risk of cancer in the United States today. JNCI 1981 (66):1130-1308

2   Higginson J: Existing risks for cancer. In: Deisler P (ed) Reducing the Carcinogenic Risks in Industry. Dekker, New York 1984, pp 1-20

3   Gough M: Estimating cancer mortality. Environ Sci Technol 1989 (23):925-930

4   Anderson EL, and the Carcinogen Assessment Group: Quantitative approaches in use to assess cancer risk. Risk Analysis 1983 (3):277-295

5   US Environmental Protection Agency: Cancer Risk from Outdoor Exposure to Air Toxics, External Review Draft. Research Triangle Park, North Carolina, 1989

6   US Environmental Protection Agency: Unfinished Business: A Comparative Assessment of Environmental Problems, Appendix I: Report of the Cancer Risk Work Group, 1987

7   Aksoy M: Benzene Carcinogenicity. CRC Press, Boca Raton, FL, 1988

8   Vigliani EC and Saita G: Benzene and leukemia. New Engl J Med 1964 (271):872-876.

9   Ott GM et al: Mortality among individuals occupationally exposed to benzene. Arch Environ Health 1978 (33):3-10

10 Rinsky RA et al: Benzene and leukemia: An epidemiological risk assessment. New Engl J Med 1987 (316):1044-1049

11 Graham JD, Green LC, and Roberts MJ: In Search of Safety: Chemicals and Cancer Risk. Harvard University Press, Cambridge, MA 1988 p 163

12 Cronkite E: Chemical leukemogenesis: Benzene as a model. Sem Hematol 1987 (24):2-11

13 Irons RD (ed) Toxicology of the Blood and Bone Marrow. Raven Press, New York 1985

14 Thorslund TW et al: Quantitative Re-evaluation of the Human Leukemia Risk Associated with Inhalation Exposure to Benzene. Final Report, Clement Associates, Inc, Fairfax, VA, October 1988

15 Goldstein BD: Clinical hematotoxicity of benzene. In: Mehlman MA (ed) Benzene: Occupational and Environmental Hazards - Scientific Update. Princeton Scientific Publishing Co, Princeton, NJ, 1989

16 Kerns WD et al: Carcinogenicity of formaldehyde in rats and mice after long-term inhalation exposure. Cancer Res 1983 (43):4382-4392

17 Sielken RL: The capabilities, sensitivity, pitfalls, and future of quantitative risk assessment. In: McColl RS (ed) Environmental Health Risks: Assessment and Management. University of Waterloo Press, Ontario, Canada, 1987

18 Crouch E and Wilson R: Interspecies comparison of carcinogenic potency. J Toxicol Environ Health 1978 (5):1095-1118

19 Starr TB, and Buck RD: The importance of delivered dose in estimating low-dose cancer risk from inhalation. Fund Appl Toxicol 1984 (4):740-753

20 Hawkins N and Graham JD: Expert scientific judgement and cancer risk assessment: A case study of pharmacokinetic data. Risk Analysis 1988 (8):615-625

21 US Dept of Labor: Occupational Exposure to Formaldehyde. Federal Register 1985 (50): 50458+

22 Wolff SK, et al: Choice of experimental data for use in quantitative risk assessment: An expert-judgement approach. J Toxicol Industrial Health 1990 (in press)

23 Graham JD and Holtgrave D: Coke Oven Emissions: A Case Study of Technology-Forcing Regulation. Report to the US Congressional Research Service, Washington, DC, 21 April 1989

24 Rosenthal A, Sawey MJ and Graham JD: Incinerating Municipal Solid Waste: A Health Benefit Analysis of Controlling Emissions. Report to the US Congressional Research Service, Washington, DC, 21 April 1989

25 Anderson FA: Environmental Improvement Through Economic Incentives. Resources for the Future, Washington, DC, 1977 pp 21-38

26 Crandall RW: Controlling Industrial Pollution. Brookings Institution, Washington, DC 1983

27 Copeland G, Associate, Temple, Barkin and Sloane, Inc, Letter to John D. Graham, 5 October 1989

28 Thompson MS: Benefit-Cost Analysis for Program Evaluation. Sage, New York 1980 pp 221-249

29 White LJ: The Regulation of Air Pollutant Emissions from Motor Vehicles. AEI, Washington, DC, 1982 p 85

30 US EPA: Evaluation of Air Pollution Regulatory Strategies for the Gasoline Marketing Industry. Washington, DC, July 1984; updated, 1988

31 Health Effects Institute: Gasoline Vapor and Human Cancer. Cambridge, MA 1985; supplement, 1988

Concluding Remarks*

1. Environmental pollution is certainly not a new phenomenon, but has substantially increased in recent times since man-made sources were added that exceeded the natural sources in importance. Air pollution is one of the main contributors to general pollution. Its components have changed over the years according to the prevailing role of their sources, and thus, while they previously originated mainly from volcanoes, wood and, later, coal burning, in more recent times the burning of other fossil fuels, a number of industrial emissions and car exhausts have been added.

2. Industrial countries, and, to a much lesser extent, developing countries, are introducing an increasing quantity of organic and inorganic pollutants into the atmosphere. A number of these pollutants have regional and global consequences, examples of which are acid rain, ozone depletion, the greenhouse effect and the ubiquitous spread of various man-made chemicals into the environment and into human tissues.

3. In this volume, special attention has been paid to outdoor pollution. It is clear, however, that not only does outdoor pollution not stop at the house door, but outdoor and indoor pollution can hardly be considered separately. In some instances, indoor pollution exceeds outdoor pollution and the fact that in most industrialised countries people spend more time indoors than outdoors should not be overlooked. It should also not be overlooked that the most important source of air pollution, namely tobacco smoke, may occur outdoors as well as indoors and may concern, with varying intensity, active as well as passive smokers.

4. Fossil fuel combustion is the principal source of pollutants of health concern (e.g., aliphatic and aromatic hydrocarbons, polycyclic hydrocarbons, SOx, NOx and metals). Several recognised human carcinogens are important air pollutants. Additional pollutants are produced as a result of many chemical, photochemical and physical atmospheric interactions. Experimental studies provide sufficient evidence that over 50 air pollutants, including a number of mixtures, are carcinogenic to animals. Efforts have been made to combine exposure data with cancer potency to estimate which air pollutants are of greatest potential risk. This analysis suggests that mixtures of incomplete combustion products account for the greatest potential risk. Air pollutants which this analysis suggests should be of concern include other chemicals which are also emitted as combustion products (e.g., 1,3-butadiene, benzene and formaldehyde), as well as Cr (VI), chloroform, asbestos, arsenic, ethylene dibromide (EDB) and dioxin. There are over 2,000 air pollutants that have not been studied in experimental systems. Many of these are present in trace quantities in the air. Complex mixtures of urban air particles and gaseous air pollutants are also mutagenic in short-term bioassays and this

---

* These remarks have been jointly prepared by all the authors of the monograph

mutagenicity in some cases increases as a result of atmospheric transformation and the formation of new compounds.

5. Epidemiological evidence suggests that urban air pollution and exposure near some types of industries may be related to an increased risk of lung cancer. The nature of the so-called urban factor has not been precisely clarified, but it cannot be identified entirely with the habit of smoking which occurred earlier and is more widespread in the cities than in the country. An increased lung cancer risk persists, in fact, even after careful adjustment for smoking. Occupational exposures, which, at least until recently, were more common in urban than in rural districts, may explain only part of the observed difference in risk.

6. Smoking-standardised excess relative risks of lung cancer in urban areas are generally in the order of 50% or less. This implies that up to one-third of the lung cancers in urban areas are related to living in such areas. The fraction that may be attributed to air pollution exposure is difficult to assess, but it is probably in the order of 5-20% of the 50% urban excess. Some support for these quantitative estimates is provided by extrapolations from findings in studies on occupational exposures.

7. The epidemiological studies on urban air pollution and lung cancer give results on the type of interaction with tobacco smoking that are somewhat inconsistent. However, most studies point to an interaction in excess of an additive effect. It is at least possible that interactions between various components of the mixture of pollutants in urban and industrial areas, both of synergistic and antagonistic nature, are of importance. On the whole, the levels of exposure to most known carcinogenic and/or mutagenic air pollutants are considerably higher in urban than in rural atmospheres. Radon and some polycyclic hydrocarbons might be exceptions in semi-rural areas where wood burning and individual heating are widespread.

8. Urban/rural differences in cancer rates are often seen for sites other than lung, but the effects are generally less pronounced. The role of air pollutants for these findings is at present impossible to assess.

9. In 1989, 86 countries declared their intention to phase out their production and use of ozone-destroying CFCs by the year 2000. In several industrialised countries, there has recently been a significant reduction in the use of leaded petrol combined with the introduction of catalytic converters and a reduction of high sulphur fossil fuels. These are just some minor signs of a common desire to reduce air pollution. A radical change in the choice of priorities in world policy and world economy would be required in order to adequately address the global environment. Since pollution control is often costly and resources are limited, decision makers should examine the relative costs and effectiveness of alternative pollution control stategies. The method of cost-effectiveness analysis can assist decision makers in using resources widely. Policy tools, such as emission fees and marketable emission permits, may be considered to enhance the cost-effectiveness of pollution control programmes. Such tools must, however, be implemented in a way that does not compromise the achievement of public health objectives.

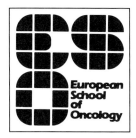

ESO Monographs
Series Editor: U. Veronesi

S. Monfardini, Aviano (Ed.)

The Management of Non-Hodgkin's Lymphomas in Europe

1990. VIII, 92 pp. 13 figs. 12 tabs. Softcover DM 84,–
ISBN 3-540-52297-2

J. C. Holland, New York; **R. Zittoun,** Paris (Eds.)

Psychosocial Aspects of Oncology

1990. VIII, 142 pp. 3 figs. Hardcover DM 82,–
ISBN 3-540-51947-5

A. Breit, Technical University of Munich (Ed.-in-Chief)

Magnetic Resonance in Oncology

A. L. Baert, R. Felix, R. Musumeci, W. Semmler and G. Sze (Co-Eds.)
1990. XIII, 173 pp. 147 figs. 7 tabs. Hardcover DM 178,–
ISBN 3-540-51054-0

A. B. Miller, Toronto, Ont. (Ed.)

Diet and the Aetiology of Cancer

1989. VII, 73 pp. 2 figs. Hardcover DM 92,–
ISBN 3-540-50681-0

F. Cavalli, Bellinzona (Ed.)

Endocrine Therapy of Breast Cancer III

1989. VII, 65 pp. 26 figs. 7 tabs. Hardcover DM 64,–
ISBN 3-540-50819-8

L. Domellöf, Örebro (Ed.)

Drug Delivery in Cancer Treatment II

Symptom Control, Cytokines, Chemotherapy
1989. VII, 107 pp. 31 figs. Hardcover DM 136,–
ISBN 3-540-51055-9

L. Denis, Antwerpen (Ed.)

The Medical Management of Prostate Cancer

1988. IX, 98 pp. 8 figs. Hardcover DM 82,–
ISBN 3-540-18627-1

B. Winograd, Amsterdam; **M. Peckham,** London; **H. M. Pinedo,** Amsterdam (Eds.)

Human Tumour Xenografts in Anticancer Drug Development

1988. XV, 143 pp. 37 figs. Hardcover DM 116,–
ISBN 3-540-18638-7

Also available:

L. Domellöf, Örebro (Ed.)

Drug Delivery in Cancer Treatment

1987. VII, 99 pp. Hardcover DM 82,– ISBN 3-540-18459-7

J. F. Smyth, Edinburgh (Ed.)

Interferons in Oncology

Current Status and Future Directions
1987. VII, 70 pp. Hardcover DM 48,– ISBN 3-540-18019-2

F. Cavalli, Bellinzona (Ed.)

Endocrine Therapy of Breast Cancer

Concepts and Strategies
1986. VII, 120 pp. Hardcover DM 46,– ISBN 3-540-16959-8

R. Mertelsmann, Freiburg (Ed.)

Lymphohaematopoietic Growth Factors in Cancer Therapy

1990. VII, 90 pp. 8 figs. 14 tabs. Hardcover DM 78,–
ISBN 3-540-53086-X

E. J. Freireich, University of Texas (Ed.)

New Approaches to the Treatment of Leukaemia

1990. VII, 193 pp. 37 figs. Hardcover DM 148,–
ISBN 3-540-52261-1

A. Goldhirsch, Lugano (Ed.)

Endocrine Therapy of Breast Cancer IV

1990. VIII, 97 pp. 19 figs. 40 tabs. Hardcover DM 68,–
ISBN 3-540-52961-6

L. Domellöf, Örebro (Ed.)

Drug Delivery in Cancer Treatment III

Home Care Symptom Control, Economy, Brain Tumors
1990. VIII, 125 pp. 34 figs. 38 tabs.
Hardcover DM 148,–
ISBN 3-540-52951-9

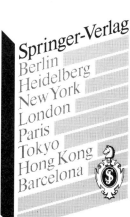

Springer-Verlag
Berlin
Heidelberg
New York
London
Paris
Tokyo
Hong Kong
Barcelona

U. Veronesi (Editor-in-Chief); **B. Arnesjø, I. Burn, L. Denis, F. Mazzeo** (Co-Editors)

Surgical Oncology

A European Handbook

Foreword by I. Burn

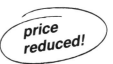
price reduced!

1989. XVIII, 999 pp. 222 figs. 227 tabs. Hardcover DM 198,–
ISBN 3-540-17770-1

… it offers instruction in the fundamental principles which underlie the essentially interdisciplinary nature of tumor surgery, and provides an excellent survey of the other nonsurgical treatment modalities.

The editors of the European Handbook of Surgical Oncology have pursued this design in a consistent fashion. In short, informative, and in most cases readily understandable chapters, the reader is first introduced to the "Biology of Cancer", "Detection and Diagnosis", and the "General Concepts in Cancer Treatment". Particularly worthwhile is the section on "General Concepts in Cancer Treatment", which succeeds in making such interdisciplinary areas as "Radiation Oncology", "Medical Oncology", "Hormones in Cancer Treatment", "Immunotherapy", as well as the "Psychological Aspects of Surgical Oncology" comprehensible to the oncologic surgeon.

The surgeon is increasingly confronted with surgical emergencies in tumor patients. The section "Emergencies in Cancer Disease", which is devoted to this problem, provides a clear overview of the appropriate emergency surgical procedures. In the section entitled "Rehabilitation Procedures", various techniques for the operative rehabilitation of tumor patients are described, particularly with respect to the special areas of plastic and orthopedic surgery. It is essential in modern oncologic practice that the therapeutic effects of multidisciplinary treatments be evaluated within the framework of controlled clinical trials. This represents the only precise method for assessment of value of various elements within a complex treatment program. "Planning and Evaluation of Cancer Treatment", the section devoted to this problem, contains, among other things, a short but nonetheless clear chapter explaining to the non-statistician the methods commonly used for analysis of recurrence and survival data.

The second half of this comprehensive volume is devoted to organ-specific tumor therapy. Again here, the interdisciplinary treatment possibilities are gone into thoroughly in each chapter…

Annals of Oncology

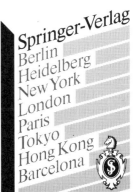

Springer-Verlag
Berlin
Heidelberg
New York
London
Paris
Tokyo
Hong Kong
Barcelona

Distribution rights for Japan: Maruzen Company, Tokyo

Prices are subject to change without notice.